PANIC AT

CALMING
THE
STORM

A JOURNEY OF HOPE
IN A WORLD OF ANXIETY

BRIAN LUDWIG

WESTBOW
PRESS®
A DIVISION OF THOMAS NELSON
& ZONDERVAN

WestBow Press books may be ordered through booksellers or by contacting:

WestBow Press
A Division of Thomas Nelson & Zondervan
1663 Liberty Drive
Bloomington, IN 47403
www.westbowpress.com
1 (866) 928-1240

ISBN: 978-1-9736-6597-7 (sc)
ISBN: 978-1-9736-6598-4 (hc)
ISBN: 978-1-9736-6596-0 (e)

Library of Congress Control Number: 2019907764

Print information available on the last page.

WestBow Press rev. date: 10/21/2019

CONTENTS

JOURNEY 1
MY STORY – PANIC ATTACKS

FIGHTING BACK FIGHTING FEAR

FOREWORD

After casually knowing Brian for less than a year, he pulled me aside and handed me a rough draft of the book. He had written it years ago; it had sat on a shelf, worn and stapled together. "Seeing you're a nurse, could you read this and tell me what you think?" he asked. Upon starting to read the manuscript, the first thing I asked myself was - Brian had panic attacks? It was hard to wrap my head around this concept. There was nothing about him that even whispered that he had once suffered greatly from an anxiety disorder.

He had approached me at the end of a Bible study held at my house. I knew him only as a great teacher and counselor. As I read the manuscript, I was so enthralled with the content that I finished it that night. The original draft encompassed only his journey with panic attacks.

Early the next day, I contacted him and said, "Brian, you have to finish this and get it published. It could help so many people!"

People suffering from panic attacks and anxiety disorders were approaching him, seeking help. They wanted to obtain the same freedom Brian enjoys. They sought answers to obtain the key to his success, and they wanted in. He would share this "crude" copy of the book with them, and he counseled them so they could live fulfilling, productive lives without anxiety.

This is how our quest began two years ago to complete the book he had started back around the year 2000.

As a nurse educator, it has always been my desire to help others. Millions suffer from anxiety disorders; many of which are undiagnosed. During the throes of panic attacks, depression, and other mental torment, individuals just want a way out and often see no hope, and solutions seem too difficult to obtain. His solutions were so easy to explain. I started sharing them with people I know. People were able to grasp the concepts easily because of his true-life analogies.

As I am an avid reader and writer, Brian asked if I would be a content consultant. Taking this on was a blessing: as a nurse to help others and as a Christian to help him organize all that God had started to reveal. During the past two years, of completing PANIC ATTACKS – CALMING THE STORM, Brian was led by Holy Spirit to add the second journey: to obtain freedom from spiritual confusion.

Karen DiGiulio, RN Nurse Educator

INTRODUCTION

Current estimates indicate that anxiety disorders affect 40 million adults in the US, while panic disorder affects up to six million people. The actual number is much higher because many have not been diagnosed. Many of the individuals who face these challenges every day do not understand how the body systems work together, so when they face the sheer terror of a panic attack, they believe they are going to die. They live their life in the dark with no hope.

Is this you or someone you know? PANIC ATTACKS – CALMING THE STORM provides important tools for anyone dealing with anxiety issues or panic attacks. The reader joins Brian as he battles to loosen the stranglehold anxiety placed on his life and regain the joy of everyday living.

Message from the author

If only a book like this, had been around when I was battling panic attacks! If I knew then what I know now I would not have gone through years of torment. The experience, as horrible as it was, has blessed me with the ability to be a blessing to others. I do not like to see others in such torment!

Brian Ludwig

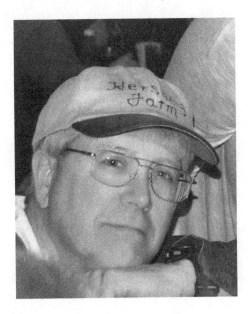

My Story – Panic Attacks

WHAT IN THE WORLD IS HAPPENING?

It was Friday, May 16, and I was hard at work. Of course, coming from a long line of workaholics, that's just the way I'm wired. Being in the restaurant business, I had an endless source of tasks to supply my addiction to work. As the operations manager of five restaurants, I was conditioned to handle pressure and successfully endured more than my share of stress. However, I enjoyed my job and felt I was able to maintain an acceptable balance. People knew me as organized, competent, and for staying rather calm in a crisis. I was always totally involved in my work, but, unlike a lot of people, when it was time to quit, I could enjoy my free time with little lingering luggage from my job. Basically, what I am saying is that, for the most part, I felt well in control of my emotions, my responses, and the general circumstances of life.

On that afternoon in May 1992, I was in my office finishing up some last-minute paperwork before starting my rounds of inspections of the restaurants, which I did several times a week. My round-trip to the five restaurants took between six to eight hours and covered about 270 miles, logged on the highways and turnpikes between two states.

On that particular Friday, I found myself experiencing some unusually uptight and tense feelings. The entire week had been pretty hard, so I attributed my uneasiness to stress. Things were going fairly well at the restaurants, so I decided to forgo the inspections and just take it easy for the evening. After a quick phone call to my restaurant managers to let them know that I would see them the next day instead of that evening, it was time to go home. I had worked enough; I would call it a day.

By all measures, this game plan should have helped me to relax and unwind. I noticed, however, that the uncomfortable feelings did not subside; in fact, if anything, they steadily increased. I decided to take a walk outside in the fresh air. That was always a good tool for helping me relax, but again, no change. I felt a strange, unaccustomed fear creeping over me. I had a headache, my breathing was fast and shallow, and I could feel each beat of my pounding heart.

At this point, I became really concerned, and my uneasiness grew to a panic. I noticed my lips beginning to grow numb, and a tingling feeling spread through my arms and fingers. *Well, that's it. Something is definitely wrong. A stroke?* I wondered. Well, I wasn't going to wait around to find out. I hopped into my truck and headed for the medical center in my hometown. The 20-minute drive was extremely uncomfortable, but at least I knew I would soon be where people could help me.

As I marched into the waiting room, I begin to relax slightly, thinking that now I would get some answers. Anxiously, I walked up to the receptionist, explained how badly I felt, and stated that I needed to see a doctor. She said they would do their best to work me in and asked me to have a seat. After sitting for only a minute or two, the same symptoms flooded over me again, only this time with renewed fury. I returned to the receptionist with a strong sense of urgency all over my face as I insisted fearfully, "I need to see someone now!"

She hurried me back to the emergency area and summoned a doctor. As a nurse tried to make me comfortable, she asked me what I was feeling. I remember explaining that I felt as if I was going to explode.

"Well, we'll just take your blood pressure," she said calmly and sweetly. She began the process, and I was handling things pretty well until I heard her reaction to the results.

"Oh, my!" she blurted as her eyes widened. Well, she didn't have to tell me. To this day, I swear I could see the mercury spurting out of the top of the gauge, just like you see on those old cartoons. What was the reading? Oh, I don't know, something like 195/whatever it was, I could tell from her reaction that the reading wasn't pretty. My heart was racing and the only thought I could muster was, "We've got problems!"

Well, the nurse hurriedly summoned the doctor. He walked in, took one look at me, and immediately told me to lie down and try to relax. *Brilliant*, I thought, *just relax. In what year of medical school did you achieve that tidbit of medical genius?* I might have been going out of my mind, but at least I was maintaining a healthy level of sarcasm.

Well, slowly but surely (definitely more slowly than surely), I began to relax. My blood pressure lowered to the point where they no longer worried that my neck would be a launching pad for my body to hurl my head into orbit like a cork on a cheap bottle of Champagne. Now we could finally get down to finding some explanations as to what had happened to me. I had never felt that way before, and I never wanted to feel that way again. After some lengthy discussions, the doctor explained that I'd had an anxiety attack brought on by consistently high levels of stress and too much work. He suggested that I take it easy for a few days, increase my physical exercise, and avoid all caffeine. This all sounded good, but I couldn't help feeling there was more to this whole thing. *Surely, there must be some medication I can take in case it ever happens again*, I thought to myself, but at this point, I was ready to accept the diagnosis and take his advice on the solution.

When I got home, I remember sitting down in my chair gingerly as if my pockets were filled with nitroglycerin. I tried to relax, ate a little something, and later in the evening, I ran for a mile and lifted some weights. I had always exercised regularly, but now I was going to take it very seriously. That night I fell asleep without too much trouble. I felt exhausted after all I had been through.

The next day, I began to feel cautiously optimistic that everything was going to be all right. I went to work as usual but decided to reduce my workload for a week or so. A few more days passed, and I continued to feel better. But something had definitely changed, for however much I tried, I just couldn't regain the carefree, relaxed nature that I used to have. I found myself almost afraid to enter into any high-pressured situation since I so vividly remembered what I had just been through. Also, I found it hard to fall asleep, which had never been a problem before. I felt boxed in when I was inside. A few nights, I ended up sleeping outside on a lawn chair. It seemed like the only place I could relax. There were just enough distinct, distant noises out there to take my mind off the way I felt, which allowed me to slowly drift off to sleep.

Time slowly passed. The exercise and slight reduction in my workload seem to bring this whole thing under fairly good control; at least it was tolerable.

Now that I look back, there were a few subtle warning signs that started to show up, but they were not frequent enough or strong enough for me to pay much attention to. I remember having headaches more often and would get tired much faster. I tended to avoid a lot of heavy mental work because I didn't always seem to have a clear head. Strangely, while driving, I would find myself hugging the edge of the road. I would position myself on the shoulder to put more distance between me and any oncoming traffic. And it wasn't just that; I also felt very uncomfortable driving down steep hills. How odd that it never bothered me before. I used to love traveling on mountain roads with steep inclines and declines, but not anymore. It even got to the point when driving itself became quite uncomfortable. Things I used to enjoy doing somehow lost their enjoyment. As you read this, I'm sure you can identify with what I'm talking about: that I felt compelled to stay near home—a place where I could decide to flee any uncomfortable circumstance immediately and retreat into familiar territory. If not, I would become even more uneasy. I needed to be in control.

From time to time, as I share my story with you, I will interject specific details about how I was feeling. It is very important that you see parallels in what I went through and what you're going through. It's very important that you identify patterns. The more you can relate to my experience, the more confidence you will begin to gain to find your way to freedom.

Anyway, I now found myself overanalyzing the things I used to give absolutely no thought to. In fact, overanalyzing is putting it mildly. I became an artist of over-analyzation. I would overanalyze until I found myself overanalyzing about overanalyzing. It was like placing my every thought in a blender and turning it on high. Needless to say, I would often feel a little off balance, and I sometimes became downright dizzy. These feelings would not happen consistently or occur all at once. Consequently, I just decided to put up with them, thinking I would soon be back to my normal self, but it was becoming obvious that my "normal" was a thing of the past.

HEY, SOMETHING JUST ISN'T RIGHT!

By this time, it was the early part of July. It was Saturday afternoon and I had spent the morning lifting weights. My routine was to lift on Saturday mornings, Monday mornings, and Thursday evenings. I would lift with a really good friend, Eric, who lived close by. We usually traveled the 20 miles to the gym together. It was our way of staying in touch and it was always an enjoyable time. So, the day had begun innocently enough.

When I got home that Saturday after lunch, I spent about 45 minutes laying in the sun. Even though I worked inside, I was determined not to look as though I did. I could usually take a nap while lying in the sun, but on that particular day, I felt very restless. Shoving those feelings aside, I decided to get ready for work and get on my way.

On the way to work, I noticed an unusual, uneasy feeling while driving. When I reached my office, which was located in the central restaurant of the group that I supervised, the uneasy, uptight feelings continued. In fact, I really didn't feel like going inside, and I waited a bit before going into the building. At that moment, for no apparent reason, my breathing had become heavy and slightly labored. Inside, the restaurant was really busy and very hectic, which seemed to trigger an anxious, panicky type of feeling. I couldn't really identify the feeling because it wasn't something I had experienced before. It reminded me of the feeling portrayed in the movies when a person is watching himself from the outside. Things were happening—people were hustling and moving around me, all busy, all with a purpose, and I felt just like an object that didn't fit into the picture. I felt as if I were moving in slow motion while everyone scurried around me. I couldn't focus or get a handle on things, let alone flow with the crowd. I remember feeling very light-headed. It took all I could do to walk and not fall over. I would fixate on an object and try to walk there and use it to catch my balance. Things began spinning.

"Show me the door," my mind screamed. "I want out."

Somehow I made it back to my office, and I briskly closed the door behind me as if a pack of wild dogs was ready to rush into the room. I tried to remember all the things I had felt that night in May and tried to come up with some connection with the way I was feeling that particular day. I knew that my feelings in May had been those of sheer terror, based on my belief that I was having major health problems. Now, however, it was more like a general fear and uneasiness about everything. I didn't really know what to do next. I could rush off to the doctor, but what would I tell him? This feeling was not based on a physical malfunction; it was more like a state of mind, or maybe I was losing my mind. After all, I certainly felt a complete lack of control over my emotions. Basically, I was afraid, and I didn't know what I was afraid of. I knew I didn't want to go back into the hustle and bustle of the restaurant. I knew I didn't feel comfortable driving. I was sane enough to know that I couldn't simply hide out in my office for the next couple of days. What exactly was happening? Was I just plain old "losing it"? Everyone kept telling me that I was under too much stress. Maybe they were right. Maybe this had no connection with my problem in May. Perhaps it was just time to admit to myself that I was having a nervous breakdown, whatever that was.

Somehow I managed to cover my responsibilities at the restaurant for the night and then headed home. Once I got out in the open, got some fresh air, and began to drive, I felt better. I was still confused by the whole episode. My memory brought me to my mother talking about some feelings she'd experienced from time to time that slightly paralleled what

I was going through. Since my parents only lived a mile from my home, I dropped in on the way home. I explained to them what was happening to me and asked if they had any insight. They were both very helpful. My father had encountered episodes in his life when he'd felt that stress had led to some very uncomfortable anxiety attacks. However, my mother's experience seemed to match certain things that I had felt more closely. She told me how driving on divided and congested highways bothered her. More interestingly, she said that, from time to time, when sitting down to a meal, whether it was at a friend's house or at a restaurant, she would get extremely uncomfortable and would not be able to eat her meal right away. She explained that she would feel a pressured, panicky type of feeling in that situation but had no idea why it happened. Well, hey, that was a start. After we talked for about an hour, I felt much better. Even though I had been going through this off and on for over two months, I had never shared it with my parents, but now I was glad I did. They gave me good insight and made me feel better about the situation. My father suggested that I take some Dramamine to help me relax and to help me sleep. I took his advice, and the evening passed uneventfully; I was even able to get a good night's sleep.

When I woke up on Sunday morning, however, I immediately sensed those uneasy, uncomfortable feelings again. I just decided to get tough and bull my way through this. I went to work and put in a semi-productive couple of hours, but I still left work feeling as if I just had to get out of there. I dropped by my parents' house again on the way home. After a lengthy discussion, we concluded that the root of the problem was based on working too hard and long at a stressful job. We believed that, subconsciously, I was probably overwhelmed by this kind of work and my mind and body were trying to tell me that this was enough. I needed a break; after all, everything up to this point that had caused these uptight feelings seemed to revolve around work.

So, I decided to take a week off. That would help me find out if I was right or not in my evaluation of the cause. I made the appropriate arrangements to take some time off.

Sunday evening and throughout the night, I felt very calm and peaceful. Monday morning, I woke up and felt okay. I decide to lift weights with Eric as I always did on Monday mornings. After that, I would fill my day with activities that were not related to work. I got ready and began to drive to meet my friend. We always met at a designated place where we left one vehicle and drove the rest of the trip to the gym together. It was only a couple of miles from our meeting point, but that now all-too-familiar feeling of uneasiness rapidly overcame me. Suddenly my heart started pounding. I was short of breath and I felt a tingling down my legs and out my arms. What was happening? Unlike my experience in May, I knew I was fine physically. I wasn't having a heart attack, a stroke, or anything like that. I had to be losing my mind. That last mile of the drive was horrible. I was weak and shaking all over. I needed help!

Finally, after pulling into the parking spot beside my friend's car and jerking my truck to a quick stop, I got out and leaned over the hood, my breathing rapid and shallow. Eric got out of his car and asked which vehicle we wanted to take. As he got closer, he noticed I was very pale and shaky and that something was very wrong. I could see he was puzzled.

"I have no idea what is going on or what the problem is," I blurted out breathlessly. "I just know something is very wrong, and I need to know what's going on."

We stood there and talked for a few minutes until I calmed down. I hadn't talked to very many people up to this point about these feelings—this overwhelming apprehension. People would think I was crazy. However, Eric was one of my best friends, and it felt good to talk about it. It was difficult, though, to explain my irrational feelings. There was no basis for what I was experiencing. Even as I attempted to explain how I was feeling at that very moment, I could only say that I was extremely uncomfortable, uneasy, and full of feelings of panic. Yes, that was it—panic—an extreme feeling of complete terror. A feeling that things were getting away from me and the fear I would never be able to get them back again. There was absolutely no sound basis or reason why I felt this way or what caused it—this was uncharted territory. Bottom line, it felt like I was going to die in one way or another. My mind hurt so bad I believed that I was about to have a total loss of control.

It was obvious I was in no shape to lift weights. I felt that driving home by myself was doable, but my friend volunteered to follow me in case there were any problems. The drive was absolutely terrible, but I made it. After Eric left, I decided to discuss the situation with my parents once again. My father was very concerned because the problem no longer seemed to be related to work. Up to this point, we had concluded that the anxiety and the stress were entirely work induced. Now we had a whole new deck of cards, and I didn't like the game. My father made an appointment with our family doctor for that afternoon and insisted on going with me. We were headed for the doctor, and we were not leaving until we found out what was going on. Sounded good to me!

OKAY, NOW WE HAVE SOME ANSWERS

On Monday at 2:00 pm, I found myself sitting in the waiting room of the medical center. Actually, it was the pre-waiting room because you get a second waiting room after the nurses take you down one of the various back hallways into one of the little rooms. Waiting was all right with me; I was not going anywhere until I found out what was wrong.

The nurse took my blood pressure. "A little high," she said. I told her that it was nothing and that I could put the readings right off the chart. She gave me a little half-smile, trying to decide whether I was trying to be humorous or if I was a professional hypochondriac. Then she said she needed to take my pulse. I looked at the clock on the wall for 10 seconds and I gave her a pulse count of 84. This time she looked at me a little funny without the half smile. "How did you know that?" she inquired.

I explained that, for the past three days, my heart had been pounding so hard, that most of the time, I could hear each beat in my head, sort of like a nervous 16-year-old kid on his first date. I explained that I had counted 14 beats per 10 seconds and multiplied by six to give her the count for a full minute. She took the pulse herself to find out I was correct. We talked a little about what I had been going through. She ended up being very nice and comforting. I told her that I have been attacking these feelings with humor because I felt as if I was on the verge of going out of my mind. She instructed me to take my time and explain everything very carefully and accurately to Dr. Jones. She was sure he could help.

Well, that was what I was banking on. Dr. Jones was always my go-to guy for important issues. All the doctors at the medical center were excellent, but Dr. Jones was the one I knew the best. Since the trouble had begun back in May, however, I had never talked to Dr. Jones. I guess since I'd been told that the problem came from stress related to my work, I'd thought there was only one obvious thing to do. However, now I knew this was much more than stress; I was here to finally get some answers.

Dr. Jones soon arrived, and I proceeded to spend the next 30 minutes explaining everything that I had been going through for the past few months. I explained that, up to this point, doctors and everyone else kept pointing to stress and being a workaholic. I knew there had to be more to it than that. After completing my little speech, the doctor put down his little chart where he was taking notes, looked me square in the eye, and smiled.

"I know what your problem is," he said. "You had a panic attack."

"Panic attack?" I repeated. "Really? Are you sure? What is that?"

"Yes, panic attack," he replied before proceeding to explain that, simply put, a panic attack is a mental and physical reaction that causes a person to react in a frantic, panicky state, with no obvious reasons to feel that way. "In other words," he said, "if something was happening, like a mugging, for example, you would go into a hyper, excitable state. Your heart would pound. You would experience fear. You would have a rush of adrenaline, and you would be in a state of panic." He went on to explain that if one feels that way without an obvious event or circumstance to stimulate the state of panic, then that is referred to as a panic attack.

"We're not really sure what causes some people to have panic attacks," he said, "but we do know that the attack itself seems to be caused by an abnormal surge of adrenaline that is released for no apparent reason. It is normal for adrenaline to be released when a person is in a dangerous situation or anxious state. However, when people experience a panic attack during a trivial or common event, for some reason, the release of adrenaline, in turn, causes the person to feel extremely uneasy and uncomfortable. A person feels panic because of that, thus causing a panic attack."

"So, I'm not going crazy?" I asked. Needless to say, I felt so good about getting some answers.

"No," he said with a laugh. "You just feel like it."

"Okay, here we go. Tell me how to get rid of this," I uttered. I was ready to attack this situation logically, the way I attacked all situations. "Well," he said, "it's not all that simple. Not everything is known about panic attacks, and it varies somewhat between people. There is medication, though, that can greatly reduce the frequency and severity of the attacks. And, just as important, understanding why people have panic attacks is crucial to controlling them."

Well, no problem there. I was ready to find out everything possible about this ridiculous ailment and beat this thing. I knew I wasn't going to go through life feeling as I had for the past few months.

After some more discussion about what to do, Dr. Jones sent me on my way with an information sheet on panic attacks, as well as a video and a prescription that he recommended as being the best thing to help control the attacks. Well, I was ready for war. I jumped off the little paper-covered table so fast that I took a few yards of the paper with me and shook the doctor's hands so hard I could have jarred the little battery right out of his Seiko watch. I don't even remember opening the door—before I knew it, I was flying down the exit hall, dragging examining table paper behind me with a look of determination on my face that alerted the huskiest of nurses and patients to get out of my way. I had some answers, some ammunition, and a whole afternoon to regain my sanity. I was ready for the battle and I was going to win. I could see the light at the end of the tunnel.

I grabbed my father on the way out and announced we were headed for the pharmacy. I told him we had our answer and we were on our way. Neither he nor my mother had ever heard of a panic attack, but all three of us felt very comfortable in the knowledge that we finally had a handle on this thing. First of all, just knowing there was a name to this wild ailment was a tremendous comfort. If I was going to be crazy, it was nice to have an official name for it. It was also nice to know that I was not some bizarre case and that there were other people who had experienced the same feelings. After all, if I was going to end up in some sort of therapy group, I would hate to be the only one there. But second, I now had a prescription that was designed to help specifically in this area. Wow—what a bright ray of hope for fighting this so-called panic attack! The sooner I could move on from this chapter of my life, the better.

Upon arriving home, I prepared for the colossal event of taking my first dose of the medication. Dr. Jones prescribed me three tablets a day, each tablet being a half a milligram. Well, here we go. I got my little pill and my glass of spring water. The only thing missing was a drum roll and the timely clang of the symbols when the first tablet finally reached my stomach. After all, I assumed that this dramatic event would be the beginning of the end of panic attacks in my life.

I'm not sure what I expected to happen, but just the experience of going to the doctor who gave me some useful information along with a proven prescription for the ailment, had a calming effect on me. For the next few days, I found myself relatively free from the effects of any panic attacks. However, I didn't realize just how deeply the anxiety of having another panic attack was embedded in me. Dr. Jones never promised that I would not experience more panic attacks; he'd just comforted me with the hope that the prescription would reduce the frequency and the severity of the attack. I went to see Dr. Jones about every two weeks, and for the rest of the summer and the beginning of the fall, things went along quite smoothly—a little too smoothly, unfortunately. Throughout that time, I had such success over panic attacks that I let my guard down. Any awareness that I was still vulnerable to an attack was neatly tucked away. Then, towards the end of September, a panic attack hit with renewed fury, and to my dismay, I was not prepared or equipped to handle it.

CALL IN THE TROOPS! WE
NEED REINFORCEMENTS!

If you have ever had a panic attack, the one thing you know for sure is that you never want to have another one. I had already experienced several, and they had been quite severe. The problem, now that I look back, is that, up until this point, I had not learned enough about them. From July to September, things progressed rather steadily. They would come and go just as quickly. I was learning only to cope with them and was being lulled into a false sense of security. My mind could not register the depth of their impact on my life and how to combat them. As soon as they vanished, there was no way I would want to dredge up that experience again. With this naive sense of security, I began to assume that I would never be held hostage by them again. Now I was about to learn that, with panic attacks, you never want to assume!

One day towards the end of September, I planned to go to the hardware store, followed by the grocery store, as I usually did on my day off. The day started uneventfully, but at my first stop, the hardware store, I sensed an uneasy feeling while standing in the checkout line. When it was my turn to pay, I felt very pressured and stressed and quickly wrote out my check. I felt that I was holding other people up. The pace seemed fine for everyone else but not for me. Attempting to dismiss those uncomfortable feelings, the next stop was the grocery store. While buying groceries, an uncontrollable, boxed-in type of feeling came upon me suddenly.

I often find myself using the words "comfortable" and "uncomfortable" as I write; however, my reason for doing so is because they describe the mindset of a panic attack victim so clearly. In my case, I was always analyzing my comfort zone in each situation.

If you have experienced panic attacks or very high levels of anxiety, I'm sure that you are also overanalyzing everything. It's not that we demand comfort; rather, we just constantly evaluate our comfort level as a survival tactic for not facing another anxiety or panic attack. Anyway, for some reason, this store just dropped off my list of places where I felt comfortable. I wasn't sure what was bothering me, but everything became a struggle. Just maneuvering my cart through the obstacles of aisle display racks was challenging. Then there were those amazingly annoying shoppers who seem to be oblivious to the fact that people are trying to pass by them, and, of course, the in-store kiosk where people with just a little too much perk are convinced that I must sample some sort of food byproduct that I can't even identify.

I began to feel faint. I was a little dizzy. Pressing on, I started to feel actual fear creep into me. I found it hard to breathe, and my heart was pounding fast. I began to feel terror and my mind was racing. What was going on? Was I having a heart attack? Was I sick? Was I going to pass out right here in the store? That would be embarrassing. Who would help me? If I was going to die on the spot, then I might as well be close to the frozen food section so they could just throw me into one of the cabinets with the Birds Eye vegetables and Swanson TV dinners. I'm glad I can joke about it now, because back then I was in a fight for my life. Death seemed inevitable.

As is common with all panic attack victims, I began to ponder my options and looked for my eventual way of escape. At first, I decided that I could just finish up quickly and get out of there. No, that would take too long. I needed a doctor! What was I going to do? I decided just to leave my cart near the checkout line while I went outside to get some fresh air. Still feeling terrible, I was able to calm down to the point where I was pretty sure I wasn't going to die on the spot. I wandered, still uneasy, around the parking lot, until I was able to function adequately. However, that deep-seated anxious feeling would not taper off. I was shaking a little and felt weak, but I was determined to get my groceries and go home. Focusing on the task at hand, I entered the store, heading straight for my cart. I eyed up the checkout lines and darted to the one I felt was moving the fastest. One person was just finishing, and there was only one other person in front of me. *I should be able to handle that*, I thought. The first person left, and the cashier began serving the second person. For some reason, there was a snag in finishing up this customer right in front of me. By this time, someone was right behind me, and suddenly I felt trapped in "no man's land." Well, the panic began again. My heart was racing. I started shaking. I was short of breath and there was no easy way out. The plan was that as soon as I got to the cashier and handed her my money, I would tell her I was nauseous and had to leave. I would tell her just to throw the change in the bag. Finally, it was my turn. Trying to gain composure, I stoutheartedly moved forward.

Before I could carry out my little plan, she looked at me and said, "I'm really sorry for the hold-up. Didn't mean to keep you waiting."

That took me off guard, and without even thinking, I replied spontaneously, as I normally would, "Oh, that's okay. I'm not in a big hurry."

Without realizing it, I responded to some meaningless small talk with her which helped divert my mind from the way I was feeling. Although it didn't make it go away, it reduced the panic to a level of just being uncomfortable. Though still slightly unnerved, I was able to finish the transaction and head for my truck. The drive home went okay, and I made it into my house without any problems. What an experience! I needed some answers.

I went to see Dr. Jones that very evening and told him about my little adventure. He told me that he hoped the medication was going to help keep my panic attacks under control, but maybe it would be good to see a specialist. We agreed that if things didn't improve over the next few weeks, he would make an appointment for me to meet with the specialist. Things didn't improve; in fact, they deteriorated quite quickly.

I was ready to do whatever it took, even if it meant going to see a "specialist." Now, we all know that you use the word "specialist" to avoid admitting to yourself and anyone else that you have been advised to go see a "shrink"; excuse me, I mean a psychiatrist. At this point, however, I really didn't care who I was going to see. I just wanted help. So, I headed into the city to see a "specialist."

I had no idea what to expect. I had never been in a psychiatrist's office before. The first thing that I became aware of was how fluffy everything was. There were fluffy chairs, a fluffy carpet, and soft, fluffy music playing, and, of course, a fish tank with tropical fish. I don't think a psychiatrist is allowed to open an office without having a relaxing tank of fish with those little bubbles coming up from the little diver and his little treasure chest.

The walls were filled with fluffy pictures of little naked babies with wings—I guess they were supposed to be angels—and tranquil paintings of relaxing mountain scenes and soothing green meadow views. I noticed right away that they didn't have any vivid action pictures, like a cheetah chasing an antelope, just ready to lunge on the poor prey and rip out its throat, or a pack of wolves circling a fragile white-tailed deer, ready to tear the victim apart.

The reading material followed the same line of thinking. As I browsed through the magazines, I noticed they didn't carry a chronicle of the history of the worst air disasters, the life and times of Charles Manson, stories from survivors of shark attacks, or articles depicting the lives of society's worst serial killers. No, everything was very neat, very calm and tranquil, nonconfrontational, and most of all, very fluffy. There were certainly no sharp objects in the room.

By that time in my progression with panic attacks, I was at a low point. I had thought I understood them, but I didn't. I had thought I could deal with them on my own, but I couldn't. Worst of all, the value of life was beginning to slip away from me. I guess that's why, after meeting Dr. Jenkins, he asked what he could do for me, to which I replied, "I just want to be happy again." I guess my reason for using that phrase as a premise for this book is that I felt I had reached rock-bottom and this ailment had control over me. Quite frankly, it was doing a very effective job of beating me up.

Of course, in the beginning, we started reviewing everything I had experienced and how I was feeling. Dr. Jenkins knew enough about panic attacks to explain areas that I hadn't even discussed with him. Again, hearing that others have also faced the exact same problem and recovered gave me a spark of hope. I focused on every fact he could give me about panic attacks because I knew the more I understood, the faster I could obtain my victory.

As it turned out, I saw Dr. Jenkins often for almost a year. During that time, there were some key elements I learned from him. He helped me become knowledgeable about the different medications for panic attacks, and what dosages I needed to take even on panic free days. He also encouraged me not to overreact to panic attacks, and he cautioned me about falling into the trap of avoiding uncomfortable situations instead of learning to face them.

After that first year, there came a point when he didn't seem to have the time or the sensitivity to help me work through "my" questions; in fact, he sometimes seemed more interested in feeding the fish in his tank than in resolving my problems. It was like he was saying this was just the way it was going to be. While under his care, I began to feel that I was settling for ongoing treatment; however, what I really wanted was to make progress towards recovery. I finally came to the point when it was time to move on.

SHOW ME THE EXIT – I WANT OFF THE RIDE

At this point, let me tell you about the effects that the panic attacks were having on my everyday life. That is, if you can call what I was going through a "life." I was never the type of person who needed lots of people or a lot of entertainment to keep me happy. Before my panic attacks began, I was always able to enjoy life and was happy in almost every situation. I enjoyed working hard and then going home to relax, watching a little TV, and then going to sleep. Well, panic attacks robbed most of that contentment from me. I spent most of my days in a very anxious state, always wondering what was going to happen next. It became increasingly hard to feel comfortable, relaxed, or peaceful since, most the time, I was trying to answer one big question: "When will the next panic attack strike?".

Upon waking, I'd analyze how I felt. Then, throughout the day, I would become aware of the slightest abnormal feelings. I just didn't want another panic attack. That was the bottom line. As a result, my every thought became so consumed with altering my life to avoid anything that I thought could possibly trigger a panic attack. In doing this, I ended up giving up most of the things that made life worthwhile. In my pathetic situation, I was determined to beat this thing—I would not let it control my life.

A conversation with my friend Eric confirmed that. On the way home from lifting weights one day, Eric and I returned to our meeting place where we'd park our cars to carpool to the gym. Before we went our separate ways, we stood and talked for a while, watching traffic fly by while standing on a bridge over a bypass. As we watched the cars race underneath us that day, he finally spoke up and revealed how concerned he was about me. He saw how much I had changed over the last year and how I seemed to be losing control. He was a person of few words. In fact, I would often kid him that his girlfriend, now his wife, had to hold a conversation for both of them all by herself. So, he didn't say much, but that day he said to me, "This thing has really got you, hasn't it? It seems like you're getting to the point of starting to lose hope."

Thinking about how to give him a response that would demonstrate the level of anxiety associated with panic attacks, I remarked, "If anyone could just get this thing off me, I would write them a check right this minute for $10,000."

"Well," he said, "if anyone is going to beat this thing, you can. Besides, you are too proud to put up with something beating up on you and way too cheap to pay good money for something you can handle on your own."

Hardly a profound revelation, but he was right. Eric knew me well. He had worked with me for a few years in the restaurant business and watched me handle a lot of difficult situations. I handled challenges well and was always very competitive. All right, then, time to get a game plan. Besides that, when you got right down to it, I was a cheapskate, and 10 grand was a lot of money, certainly more than I had.

So, how was I going to beat this? There had already been a few steps of progress in my battle against these attacks, so my evaluation began there. I began to take more notes, highlighted my successes, and slowly began to uncover some very useful information.

For those who have never experienced a panic attack, let me take a few minutes to review my experience of how it feels. In _Level One_, you experience the onset of irrational fear in a situation that should not be threatening. The first symptom usually noticed is a very rapid heartbeat. I can explain it best by comparing it to running fast and hard for a few minutes and then stopping very quickly and just being really still. You can feel and hear each heartbeat. Well, that's how your heart feels when you have a panic attack. The difference, however, is that when you run and then stop suddenly, you know why your heart is beating like that. With a panic attack, there is nothing to explain the strange occurrence.

Next, you feel a surge coming from your chest and stomach area, which shoots down your arms and down your legs. It's like a mild electrical shock followed by a tingling sensation in your hands and feet. The best thing I can compare it to is driving on an icy road. You need to stop, but when you hit the brakes, you skid on the ice, and you don't think you're going to stop in time. When you finally come to a stop, you feel a surge of adrenaline all through your body. Or if you've never experienced that, think about what Dr. Jones told me: imagine yourself walking down a dark, abandoned street and suddenly being mugged. Or did you ever get a phone call in the middle the night, let's say from a hospital or the state police, and your first assumption was that it would be bad news? In these situations, you get a very uneasy, anxious feeling. Your heart beats loud and fast and you feel extremely tense and uneasy. You then feel a rush of adrenaline through your body, causing you to feel short of breath, weak, and often dizzy. Your heart is racing and a feeling of sheer terror envelops you. Well, basically those are the feelings you experience when a panic attack hits, and those feelings become more intense as you progress rapidly from one level of panic to the next.

In _Level Two,_ of the severity of a panic attack, the threatening physical symptoms in your body become alarming, adding a very real fear to the initial irrational fear. Additional adrenaline is released in response to the second wave of fear, which causes you to be even shorter of breath. You are incapable of thinking logically or rationally to deal with the situation; in fact, you feel yourself losing control, and sheer terror sets in.

In _Level Three,_ the severity of a panic attack is what I refer to as "meltdown" when uncontrolled panic takes over. You are convinced that all hope is gone, and you are sure you are going to die. You shake and tremble all over, you can hardly speak or breathe, and your heart is racing out of control. In some cases, it may even cause a person to faint.

Well, there you are. That's the process from the initial uneasiness to a full-blown panic attack. As horrible as it sounds, it can be controlled and eventually overcome. Contrary to how you feel, you will not die from a panic attack. However, it can ruin your life if left untreated, so it is crucial to learn how to stop an attack in its tracks.

I took some extra time to share with you the experience that I went through so that you can identify some similarities in your own experiences with panic attacks. I also briefly went over the progression of panic attacks because understanding the progression enables you to put a stop to things before they get out of control.

Your story may be slightly different than mine. Though you may suffer from anxiety attacks rather than panic attacks, the path to freedom is the same. This may be a good time to explain one of the major differences.

Panic Attack (no identifiable stressors)

Anxiety Attacks (identifiable stressors): Examples of anxiety stressors are actual situations or specific thoughts that bring on anxiety. Once you learn how to understand and gain control of your mind and thought patterns, you can learn how to alleviate the stressors.

Examples of stressors that can cause anxiety:

- Knowing finances are bad and you could lose everything
- Replaying in your mind why your spouse left you
- Documented health concerns
- Finding out someone you care about is an alcoholic or is addicted to drugs
- Fears of being alone, pain, suffering, loss, etc.

Now, let's get on to some of the fundamentals of gaining control of panic attacks. First, you need to have a good understanding of what is happening. Second, you need to regain control, and third, you must learn how to retake anything that panic attacks have been able to rob from your life.

Basic Comparison

Panic Attack
Sudden and Intense
Can peak in
10 -20 min
or run back to back...

Shared symptoms

Some shared
symptoms include

Anxiety Attack
More gradual
Symptoms may be
persistent and
long lasting

Happens without a known stressor
No identifiable cause

Increased Heart rate
Shortness of breath
Dizziness

Stressor Induced
Identifiable cause
Overwhelming anxiety feels like an attack

(Panic Attack – feelings of sheer fear and terror, thoughts
of impending doom, with many physical symptoms)
(Anxiety – excessive persisting worry, irritability, inability to calm
down, uneasiness, muscle tension and physical symptoms)

FIGHTING BACK
FIGHTING FEAR

UNDERSTANDING YOUR OPPONENT –
PREPARING FOR BATTLE

Over the years, I have helped so many people gain their freedom over panic attacks; not because of medical expertise, but because I was a victim. In the case of panic attacks and the success of overcoming panic attacks, experience definitely becomes the best teacher.

On my road to recovery, doctors were important. However, the most useful knowledge gained was from my own experiences and by talking to others who have also experienced panic attacks.

It's interesting how, when you watch the Olympics, you often see that the most successful coaches and trainers are those who have won major titles. If they did not win any titles, they would gain credibility when they trained someone who won a title or an event. I feel that with all I have been through, the experience has positioned me to be an effective coach.

Panic attacks can be so debilitating and damaging to the extent that a victim often loses all hope. My hope is that, from my personal experience and insight, my victory can be shared with others. Please don't take that as an arrogant statement; I'm just saying that experience has blessed me with the ability to be a blessing to others.

In one particular case, a victim that I was dealing with was convinced that he would never lead a normal life. He had only known me for a brief period and had started to attend one of the Bible studies I was leading. Because of this relationship, it was evident to him that I would not lie. He saw me as one who had lived with panic attacks and overcome them. With that credibility, I promised him that he would receive his freedom from panic attacks. Sometimes having the full trust of someone is crucial for them to gain their liberty. Anyway, through working closely with this person, he has now progressed to the point where he is no longer held hostage by fear, anxiety, or panic attacks. He received his freedom, and I am fully confident that you will receive your freedom also.

Here are some steps that we will follow to pave your path to freedom:

- **Insight and information – enabling you to compare your situation with mine.**
- **Comparing and discussing your suffering from panic attacks with others.**
- **Identifying patterns in your own life.**
- **Setting up a strong defense to get things under control.**
- **Going on the offensive to retake any lost ground.**
- **Maintaining freedom.**

I experienced my first panic attack in 1992. Amazingly, it seems that, back then, very little was known about this disorder. Along with that, I had no access to information over the internet like there is today.

Anyway, I remember the first time that I talked to a fellow panic attack victim. It was so amazing to note the similarities and patterns we shared. A large part of setting up our defense for you will be to know what you are and will be facing. By knowing what you are facing, it will enable us to establish a defensive plan that will keep you protected from being taken hostage by this disorder.

Okay, let's begin to get our defenses in order. From this point on, I will be giving you information that will include a spiritual insight into situations and solutions.

Ultimately, it was my faith in God that brought about my deliverance. If you do not believe in God, you will still find the information that I give you to be extremely helpful. Through your journey to obtain your freedom, it is my prayer that you find God in the process.

Whether you look at a panic attack as a spiritual or non-spiritual enemy, the bottom line is that the root of the effectiveness of a panic attack is fear.

The severity of your panic attacks will determine how drastic the measures we pursue to obtain your freedom are. For the sake of instruction, I'm going to be counseling you based on the premise that panic attacks have robbed the quality of your life and you are ready to do whatever it takes to obtain your freedom.

One thing that can be very frustrating is seeking support from people who have never struggled with anxiety or panic attacks. Whether these people are friends, relatives, or even doctors, they have a lot of trouble wrapping their heads around what you're going through and may end up classifying you as nothing more than a "stressed-out hypochondriac." Most of the time, they will try to offer a simple, rational solution to a very complex irrational situation. Oftentimes, people will say, "Well, when this feeling hits you, can't you just reason in your mind that it is just another panic attack occurrence and not overreact to it?"

Oh, if it could only be that easy.

If you are fortunate enough to have someone willing to work closely with you to help you gain your freedom, it will probably be very helpful if they also read this book. I know it was extremely helpful for my friends to be able to help once they understood.

The problem is that, even though you know you are overreacting, the slightly different circumstances of each situation will tend to mask the obvious pattern. For instance, you might have been shoveling snow, and your mind convinces you that you must have overdone it. Even something as simple as a bad case of heartburn can start the ball rolling. Once, when

I dropped something heavy on my foot and smashed my big toe, I was absolutely convinced that I was going to get a blood clot.

Remember, a panic attack can start up for no rational reason. However, people are different, so what comes first? Does the panic attack cause one to overthink and become a hypochondriac about all health issues, or does a person's personality trait of overthinking make them more susceptible to panic attacks and possibly trigger the initial Level One response? The jury's out on this one.

One of the first things you must know about panic attacks is that the war takes place in your head. What I am going to teach you in this and the upcoming chapters will be pivotal for your recovery and deliverance.

The body is amazingly complex. However, as we travel the road to your freedom, we don't have to be trained physicians or psychiatrists; we only need to know what is causing the way we feel and learn how to put a stop to it.

When we experience a panic attack, what we're dealing with is the inappropriate release of adrenaline. The release of adrenaline is a very normal and crucial body function. Strong emotions, such as fear or anger, cause adrenaline to be released into the bloodstream, which causes an increase in heart rate, muscle strength, blood pressure, and sugar metabolism. This reaction, known as the "flight or fight response," prepares the body to cope with dangerous, potentially life-threatening situations.

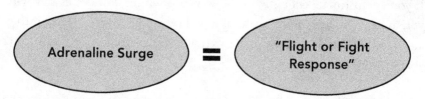

When exposed to a dangerous situation, your mind perceives impending danger. Adrenaline is released to empower you to face the danger or flee from it. This is a normal response.

If you are struggling with a panic attack, there is a logical explanation for your irrational feelings and behavior, even though the actual "Panic Attack" is illogical. For some reason, your mind and your emotions are perceiving something as being threatening to you when it isn't. This is where your subconscious comes into play. The subconscious is a part of your mind which operates without your awareness.

Okay, it is crucial that you understand this process.

In a normal situation, a person would perceive danger in their mind and in their emotions. This perceived danger would cause a release of adrenaline that would physically empower them to handle the situation. In turn, their heart would race, and they would enter a heightened awareness of a very energized state of their body. Let me give you an example. Let's say that you come home and no one else is in the house. Suddenly, you hear a loud noise in another room. You perceive danger, adrenaline is released, and that adrenaline increases your heart rate and your energy. At this point, you are energized to either flee or face a potential danger. So, in this heightened state of energy, you go into the room from which the noise came to investigate the situation. You discover that the bracket that holds a large picture on the wall came loose and the picture came crashing to the floor. As soon as the source of the apparent danger is identified, and the mind concludes that the danger is no longer present, the body relaxes, and the adrenaline flow stops because the mind has identified that there is no impending danger.

Cool process. We were created, in a way, to prepare us for danger. However, what if you entered your house and you felt exactly the same way, yet you could not attribute a reason to it?

So, you walk into the house, and suddenly you feel the effects of a release of adrenaline. Your heart starts pounding, you begin to sweat, it's hard to breathe, and you feel surges of energy racing through your body. The only problem is that there's no apparent reason for this feeling. There is no danger that we can identify. So, what's going on?

For some reason, your subconscious perceives danger. It is an irrational fear that your mind is not aware of. Without your mind being aware of what is happening, adrenaline is released into your body. I find it amazing that a perceived irrational fear in your subconscious somehow has the ability to cause a release of adrenaline. You have all the symptoms that you would experience if you were facing danger, but you are not, and unfortunately, you are unable to wrap your mind around why your body is in this heightened level of energy and awareness. In your efforts to gain an understanding, you begin to overthink the situation. "Why do I feel this way? Why is my heart pounding? Why is it hard to breathe?"

At this point, the first thing that most people conclude is that there is a major malfunction of their body and they are probably facing a heart attack, a stroke, or a mental breakdown. Because of the fear of the unknown, a second rush of adrenaline is then released into the bloodstream. This is what I refer to as a second-level panic attack. The gripping part of this situation is that now everything that you felt initially that caused you to enter into terror has now become so much worse. Everything that you felt initially that you could not understand, caused by an initial release of adrenaline, now causes your mind and emotions to react to a tangible fear, which then releases a second wave of adrenaline, thus causing the initial fear to become a present terror.

This sounds complicated, but it's not. And just to let you know, I hate using the word "subconscious" because it's not always fully understood. I'm not saying that every panic attack will initiate in the subconscious, but it definitely initiates without the awareness of the mind. If the mind was able to understand the initial reaction, there would not be a further release of adrenaline.

Now that I gave you a lengthy explanation, let's revisit the role of adrenaline.

The release of adrenaline is a normal bodily function. It's meant to protect you. In a normal situation in which you face danger, adrenaline is released, your body goes wild, you eliminate the danger, and you relax.

In the malfunction wonderfully called a panic attack, there is no apparent danger; however, something triggers a release of adrenaline into your bloodstream. Your heart races, you have trouble breathing, and you feel extremely uncomfortable because of the energy your body now experiences. Because your mind cannot grasp what is happening, it and your emotions trigger a second wave of adrenaline to be released, and your symptoms escalate to a state of panic. If things are not resolved quickly, the body can once again release adrenaline to cause what I refer to as a meltdown.

There are two issues that you often face with panic attacks.

Number one, for some reason, situations that are completely devoid of any apparent danger for an unknown reason have become dangerous or uncomfortable for you.

Number two, your mind seems to race much more than other people's. You overthink and you overanalyze. When things happen that you can't understand and bring to closure, your mind is relentlessly put to work an effort to obtain that elusive understanding. Can you relate? Oh, most definitely you can.

Within the two issues that I just referred to, there can be several side issues.

First of all, I believe some people have a stronger and a more adverse reaction to adrenaline than other people. There are people who thrive on intentional risk-taking lifestyles and dangerous behavior where death is a possibility. They intentionally seek adrenaline rushes as a form of entertainment. Just between you and me, I want to punch those kinds of people. Yeah, they love roller coasters—the bigger the better—and they may also be addictively drawn to horror flicks. So, instead of having an adverse reaction to adrenaline, these people live for it.

Secondly, some people are just much more perceptive than others. They perceive, and they overanalyze. This is the category in which I fall. I often watch my friends, who live in this bizarre state of being oblivious to almost everything that goes on around them. Nothing seems to faze them. Of course, these are those who go on a trip and their preparation is one of throwing a few things in a discarded shopping bag the morning they are scheduled to leave. In contrast, I am someone who spends days in preparation, following lists and reminders left all over the house and, of course, eventually packing two to three times more than what is really needed for the trip, often just in case someone I'm traveling with forgot something. Those oblivious people, if they would only pack what they needed instead of relying on me. Can you identify? Sure you can.

These low-key, nonchalant people are so annoying. They experience what I would classify as alarming physical conditions, and they don't even respond to them; they just assume that it is nothing and it will soon pass. One time, my friend told me that he did not feel very good on that particular day and that, around lunchtime, he got really dizzy and passed out for a few minutes. However, when he woke up scraped himself off the floor, and walked around for a while, he continued on with his day as if nothing had happened. We all know this kind of person—the kind who can slice their finger down to the bone, wrap it in electrical tape, and continue working.

Are you kidding me? What are you talking about? How do people do that? If that had been me before I learned what I know now, I would have been in the emergency room undergoing every test of my physical health that was available.

Oh well, I guess it just goes to show how different people are. Most of the time, the people I counsel and minister to who deal with panic attacks tend to be very perceptive and analytical. They are far from being oblivious, and most of the time, I would say that they fall on the side of overthinking things.

As we progress along to obtaining your freedom from anxiety and panic attacks, I will interject information like this to help you identify your personality traits and your tendencies, and even more importantly, to help you really get to know yourself, appreciate your good qualities, and laugh at your crazy ones.

Well, time's a wasting. Now that we have gained some information, let's start exploring what defenses we are going to establish to begin to get any anxiety or panic attacks that you are experiencing under control. Life is too good to waste being in fear.

To build your defense arsenal, we will examine medical insight, self-awareness, and spiritual insight in greater depth and learn how they "interconnect."

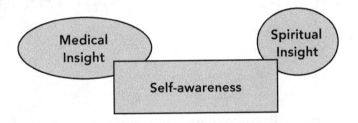

THE MIND, THE MEDS, AND THE MD

A strong defense will revolve around two main issues.

Let's review the two main conditions that you face with panic attacks:

First, for some reason, situations that are completely devoid of any apparent danger are perceived as dangerous or uncomfortable.

Second, your mind seems to race much more than other people. You overthink, and you overanalyze. When things happen that you can't understand and bring to closure, your mind is relentlessly put to work in an effort to obtain that elusive understanding.

We've already discovered a few inclinations that affect those with panic attacks.

You are consumed with thoughts about your health and safety.

Oversensitivity to adrenaline, which may affect you more than other people. Personality tendencies towards overthinking and overanalyzing situations.

You always seem to worry more about things than others do.

Next, let's explore a few other reasons why these conditions found their way to the surface.

For some reason, you have developed ruts in the patterns of your thinking and thoughts now seem to travel along familiar paths. You find it hard to change the way you think. Somehow a fear of situations and circumstances has become lodged in your subconscious without you being aware of it.

Now that we have listed a few suggestions as to why you may be vulnerable to panic attacks, let's look at behavioral reactions that I believe you are probably experiencing.

BEHAVIORAL REACTIONS

- You find it very hard to just relax.
- You are often very stressed.
- Instead of living, you feel like you have entered into a survival mode.
- Happiness has been replaced with mere toleration.
- You have established places and situations you avoid because your association with those places and situations brings about fear and discomfort.
- Your number of safe places continues to dwindle.
- Your mind is tired. You often wake up fatigued, and as the day goes on, you often feel the need for a nap.
- When you experience an unusual symptom in your body, you tend to fixate on that symptom.
- Trips are no longer fun like they used to be. They now require so much preparation and planning that the work and the stress seem to outweigh the anticipated enjoyment.
- You find yourself very uncomfortable when you are in a facility with a large number of people, especially if it is crowded.
- When you are in a strange or crowded place, you always seek out and identify ways of escape.
- You become anxious when you find yourself in a long line of people waiting for something.

- **Even on a short trip like an errand, you often find yourself taking along bottles of water and other supplies you anticipate you "may" need.**
- **Sometimes when in a crowded restaurant, you find it hard to eat.**
- **You prefer situations where you can keep your options open. You don't necessarily prefer to drive, but on the same hand, you don't feel comfortable being trapped in another persons vehicle without a way of escape.**
- **If you are in a large grocery store, or any kind of store, you begin to get more and more uncomfortable the further away you get from the exit.**
- **You find fewer and fewer situations that you look forward to.**

Wow, quite a list, but I guarantee that, if you suffer from panic attacks, you can identify with a lot of these feelings.

Okay, our defense starts with:

- ✓ Establishing your good health by choosing a qualified doctor and medications (if necessary).
- ✓ Continuing to learn about triggers that cause panic attacks and anxiety disorders, along with gaining insight into what makes you vulnerable so you can identify and reduce vulnerabilities.

Adding to this, you must:

- ✓ Learn the importance of thoughts and gaining insight into how vital it is that you learn how to control them.
- ✓ Control the way you behave by controlling the way you think.
- ✓ Grasp the importance of mental barriers and your mindset.
- ✓ Become informed that spiritual insight can be the key to your freedom. The word and promises of God are ultimately what freed me.

Our defense is aimed at procedures and resources that are geared to reducing rampant, uncontrollable fear and anxiety as a result of damaging speculation.

The definition of *fear* is "an unpleasant emotion caused by the belief that someone or something is dangerous, likely to cause pain or become a threat."

The definition of *anxiety* is "a feeling of worry, nervousness, or unease, typically about an imminent event or something with an uncertain outcome."

The definition of *speculation* is "the forming of a theory or conjecture without firm evidence."

What we are going to do is train ourselves to head off speculation before it has a chance to affect us. Speculation is the driving force behind anxiety and fear. Speculations are thought patterns that are entertained and accepted, even though there is no firm evidence of truth. From now on, we are going to learn how to demand firm evidence to dismiss the need for speculation. As we commit to only reacting to firm evidence, we will effectively reduce the negative impact of fear, panic, and anxiety in your life.

AN EFFECTIVE DOCTOR

When dealing with panic attacks, a doctor's qualifications are important; however, even more important is their commitment to helping you deal with something that, from time to time, neither you nor the doctor will be completely able to wrap your minds around.

In my case, I began with a very excellent doctor, but unfortunately, he couldn't devote the time that I felt I was going to need. The second doctor was the psychiatrist that I mentioned. I gained some good information, but I was not convinced that he was as committed to obtaining freedom as I was. His methods seemed to focus on maintaining the disorder with medications as opposed to obtaining complete freedom from the disorder.

Later, I was blessed to find Dr. Stratton, who was very sensitive and understanding. You must remember, back in 1992, panic attacks were not as well understood as they are today.

Three things told me that Dr. Stratton was a person I wanted to work with.

1. He flat out acknowledged that he did not know everything about panic attacks; however, he was very anxious to learn about the condition, which was awesome. As Dr. Stratton provided medical knowledge, I provided the hands-on experience of dealing with panic attacks. We made a great team.
2. His commitment to helping me overcome panic attacks brought me great reassurance.
3. What is perhaps most important is that, even though he never experienced a panic attack, he believed me in what I said I was going through. Because of this, he knew that I might initially have a lot of questions and concerns. He never made me feel like I was a bother to him or the least bit annoying.

Dr. Stratton's care was pivotal for me to gain control over my panic attacks. He was one of the people who suggested that it would be very helpful to others if I wrote a book about my experiences and my insights.

Because of everything that I'm sharing in this book, you do not need to find a person *exactly* like Dr. Stratton, but it is important to find a doctor who will have the initial time and patience to help you get things under control. You need to find a doctor with whom you feel comfortable, who will be sensitive to what you're going through, and who will understand your obsessive need for reassurance about your health while you are initially fighting panic attacks.

As far as your medical care, the first thing that I suggest is that you have a complete physical. I will discuss this more in the upcoming chapters. Our tactic here is to nullify the effects of speculations. Speculations run rampant when there is no evidence. To stop speculation, obtain the necessary evidence.

So, in my case, I had a complete physical done—the works. I had my heart checked out thoroughly with an EKG and a stress echo, while I also had complete blood work done and everything else they could possibly examine. I was poked and checked in areas not meant to be poked and checked. If they had given volume discounts on pricing, I would have made out great. I even had an MRI done on my brain. Now, I include this information knowing how completely I am opening myself up to cheap shots like, "Well, you surely needed to have your head examined," but I was having such severe headaches that I had to do this for my own peace of mind. I destroyed the speculation that the headaches were caused by a brain tumor by providing firm evidence that everything checked out perfectly.

Through having a complete physical, I obtained a path to again enjoying a taste of peace of mind. We were nowhere close to recovery, but there was a slight ray of hope when I was able to shut down harmful speculation. When I would start to feel something was wrong and found myself beginning to dwell on it, I could shoot down those thoughts with the ammunition of a perfect physical examination report.

> **Firm evidence disables harmful speculation.**

CORRECT MEDICATION

The prescription of correct medication is a complex and controversial subject. Some people have no trouble with the thought of medications, while others get stressed about the idea of being dependent on something.

Let me try to make this easy for you. I believe some people can obtain freedom from mild levels of anxiety and panic attacks without medication. Then there are others who are definitely going to need medication with what they're facing.

In writing this book, I tend to be targeting those people who are really struggling with anxiety and panic and whose episodes are bordering on becoming debilitating. What I mean by that is that anxiety and panic have been able to significantly influence and reduce the quality of a person's life.

Okay, for most people, I would say that medications are going to be required, but I'd also like to say that, in a lot of cases, the medications will be able to be reduced or eliminated.

For those of you who have been getting beaten up by anxiety and panic the way I was, initially, I was very thankful for the medications.

When you are constantly experiencing anxiety and panic attacks, the mind is put through a lot of stress and pressure. I like to look at it as a mind being somewhat fractured or broken, and as such, it needs time to heal.

If you break a leg, you need a cast on that leg to protect it and give it time to heal properly, to become strong again. Medications for panic attacks can be looked at in the same way.

Medications come in two forms. The first type of medication is taken for a quick fix, taken to help reduce the effects that adrenaline has on your body. The second type of medication is recommended for the long term.

So, to make it clear, medications help you reduce the harmful effect that excessive adrenaline has on you, while they also provide support for your mind—like a cast on your leg—to give it an opportunity to rest and become strong and healthy.

On our road to recovery, I strongly suggest that you get a complete physical to enable you to begin dismissing wild speculations that you are facing a life-threatening medical issue. Now, along with that, I'm suggesting that you consult with your doctor about the use of medication to reduce the effect that adrenaline has on your body and to help your mind from racing owing to your irrational catastrophic thinking.

In my case, my mind was broken. For too long, I allowed myself to get beaten up by anxiety and panic before I finally learned how to get things under control. Because of that, my mind was in this fragmented state. Because of debilitating anxiety and fear, for lack of better terminology, we will refer to your mind as being "severely bruised or broken." Just as with a broken leg, we need to get your mind and emotions to the place where healing can begin its process. We must establish an atmosphere where the frequency of fear, anxiety, and panic are greatly reduced.

When you get a complete physical exam, you take away the fuel that your mind feeds on to race. Again, what we're doing is establishing a defense against speculation. Remember, the definition of speculation is "the forming of a theory or conjecture without firm evidence." When we have had a complete physical and have received a clean bill of health, harmful speculations are drastically reduced. Then it's time to improve the strength of your mind by giving it some support from needed medications.

For those of us who are committed to learning to live by faith in God, taking medications may seem to be contrary to that. I will address this later in the book, but first, let me make two points. If I'm going to take medications, I'm going to take medications in faith. I pray over the medications, and I believe they will be effective. Also, through my journey of dealing with anxiety and panic attacks, I've learned so much spiritually that I did not know before. In being able to share this with you, my prayer is that it will hopefully be a major part of your deliverance, as it was with me.

For me, because of these benefits, my mind and body found it a lot more difficult to conspire together to send me into a fit of terror. When I was feeling something wrong in my body, I developed a much stronger positive response to potentially troubling symptoms.

My out-loud response was, "No, I just had a complete physical. You are overreacting, being too sensitive. Now, shut up and behave yourself."

Now, don't get me wrong, if you have an actual physical problem, you must use good judgment. However, just as important is that you must not let your vulnerability to fear and panic cause you to have what I call a mental monopoly on hysteric hypochondria. What worked best for me was to have regular checkups with Dr. Stratton every two weeks during the initial recovery time. That way, we could discuss my progress, and it kept me from running to see him every time I felt bad. I could just tell myself that my appointment was coming up and that I'd be fine until then. Looking back, it sounds so easy. But when you are afflicted by panic attacks, hardly a day passes without you feeling the need to go to a doctor. You just feel so bad that you think you must have some help for that day. But trust me, if you're in that state, the steps we are taking will effectively put you on the road to recovery and freedom.

So, our first steps are finding a sensitive competent doctor, getting a complete physical, and using the necessary medications to help in the initial healing process. A good doctor and correct medication are extremely important. However, I believe what we're going to learn in the next chapters will be pivotal to getting things under control.

Doctors and medication are great, but I didn't want to be dependent on them for the rest of my life, and I'm sure you don't either.

What I'm going to tell you next is essential.

One of the most important things to obtain in the state that you're in is the success of getting through a day without getting beaten up by anxiety and panic. The next most important thing is to begin to string a few days back to back to where you actually begin to experience some normality in your life.

As we continue to establish your defense, we will now focus on gaining even more information on panic attacks and how to deal with them. In the following chapters, we will focus on what you, as a victim, can do to obtain your freedom.

DISSECTING FEAR, ANXIETY, AND SPECULATION

Anxiety is living life constantly prepared to fail and continually rehearsing how you will cope with the impending failure.

The initial phase of the defense that we set up involves professional medical help and medications. Both are important in the beginning, but it is my opinion that your ultimate freedom is going to be found by gaining more and more knowledge of what is going on that creates anxiety and panic. Also, we will learn how vital it is to receive help from others.

Remember, a doctor is very important to verify that you are in a good state of health. It was amazing to me how horrible I often felt even though I was perfectly healthy. Whether you rely on a doctor to treat you for your panic attacks is a decision that you will have to make. However, if the panic attacks are severe and if you often are obsessed with fear concerning your health, I feel it is essential to obtain a complete physical, as I discussed before. Make a yearly physical a must.

Also, medications can be important as a type of "cast" for something that is severely bruised or broken; in this case, that would be your mind.

I have successfully helped people who have relied on doctors and medication, and I have successfully helped people who choose to fight it on their own with the help of non-professionals. You will know the right decision for you.

Having said that, your path to freedom is going to be found in the next chapters. This is a part that I enjoy so much; that is, sharing information with people that enables them to obtain their freedom. So, buckle up, and let's go rescue your life and bring it back to a place of peace, joy, and contentment.

You will notice that, through the next several chapters, you will be provided with more and more information. Some information, you will begin to grasp immediately. Some information, you will only be able to adopt after a foundation has been established. Repetitious information will help it become ingrained. Providing repeated information that may come at you in slightly different ways will also help you form a foundation so that, when it comes the time for you to take action, you will be fully prepared to do it effectively.

The basis of anxiety and panic attacks is fear. Fear has the ability to lie to you. Think of how many times you entertained fear only to later find that there was no basis for that fear.

When you are very vulnerable to fear, it will be very effective at lying to you. If you had a friend who lied to you as much as fear lies to you, that friend would very quickly lose their "friend" status with you. For the record, we're going to identify fear as your enemy, your tormentor.

The definition of *fear* is "an unpleasant emotion caused by the belief that someone or something is dangerous, likely to cause pain or become a threat."

The definition of *anxiety* is "a feeling of worry, nervousness, or unease, typically about an imminent event or something with an uncertain outcome."

The definition of *speculation* is "the forming of a theory or conjecture without firm evidence."

We are going to obtain your freedom through exposing, and finally obtaining victory over, fear, anxiety, and speculation. As we deal with speculation, we will gain more insight into reasonings and into your imagination.

You can see from the above-mentioned definitions how fear, anxiety, and speculations work together to torment you.

When you are a victim of panic disorder, you seem to be in a constant state of nervousness and unease. You aren't always sure why, but most the time you are nervous and very uncomfortable. Okay, let's figure out why.

Fear is tormenting; fear is an unpleasant emotion. Somehow a thought pattern has been established where you perceive possible danger, pain, or loss. Since there is no firm evidence, what you perceive has come in the form of speculation. Speculation is the attempt to draw a conclusion without firm evidence. As we learned before, the perception of fear causes a release of adrenaline into your bloodstream. When you are in fear because of obvious danger, the presence of adrenaline provides energy to deal with that danger.

FACE TO FACE WITH A BEAR

Once, while spending time at my cabin in the mountains, I came out the door of the cabin onto the deck and down a flight of stairs that led to the yard. As I walked through the yard to the edge of the cabin, I came face to face with a large black bear. I wasn't quite prepared for that, and I'm not sure which one of us was the most startled, but I had no plans of staying around to see what was about to happen. Adrenaline shot through my body, and I found myself energized for action. I realized this because the number of steps it took to come out of the cabin, onto the deck, down the stairs into the yard, and into the presence of my unexpected guest were many more than the few steps it took me to get to the cabin door to reach a place of safety. In fact, I'm not even sure if I even used the steps; I just remember catapulting myself from the yard to the cabin door. That's the blessing of adrenaline. Adrenaline empowers you with energy to either fight the danger or flee from the danger. I don't mind telling you that, in this case, the decision of whether to fight or flee was not lengthy or labored.

Once in the cabin, in my place of safety, the adrenaline rush quickly dissipated, and it was enjoyable watching the large bear stroll through our yard, into the woods, and then up the side of the mountain. So, I came face to face with danger, identified the danger, and intelligently removed my presence from the danger. In doing so, I watched the danger go away, and I no longer perceived it as being a danger.

Okay, this is huge. Adrenaline is released when there is a perceived danger. Unfortunately, if you enter into fear based on speculation (i.e., theories instead of facts), adrenaline will be released into your bloodstream and there will be an increased heartbeat and a lot of energy. Your body is being prepared to fight or flee the danger. Often, the subconscious will initiate fear, and the mind will receive it as speculation. This is where the problem lies.

When you are dealing with fear rooted in the subconscious and based on speculation, you cannot identify the source of the fear. Therefore, you cannot identify why you are in fear, so...

It will be impossible for you
to know when you are no longer
in a place of danger!

In the case of the bear, we met, I didn't like it, I identified the danger, I felt fear, I fled from the danger, I perceived safety, and the fear dissipated.

Panic attacks are based on fear without a danger that can be identified. Either you cannot identify the danger or, in a lot of cases, what you perceive as being dangerous or uncomfortable is only dangerous and uncomfortable in your mind.

> ## THIS IS BIG!
>
> **When you feel fear but you are unable to identify the danger, there is no way to identify when the danger is gone, so you are held captive by ongoing fear that you do not have the ability to stop.**
>
> **Speculation initiates fear, and fear fuels speculation.**

Fear is an unpleasant emotion caused by the belief that something is dangerous or threatening. Speculation is the forming of a conclusion based on a theory that has no firm evidence.

Here we go—fear is very unpleasant for anyone who suffers from panic attacks. Because of that, you become overly watchful. Instead of being in a relaxed state, you are anxious and live with constant anxiety. Because of that, your nerves become what the medical field labels as being in a state of "sensitization." What this means is that your nerves and your feelings are in a much more heightened state of awareness than the average person. If you are in a state of nerve sensitization, it's very important to understand that the effects of adrenaline on your body will be much more severe than for someone who mostly operates in a very calm and peaceful state. This is why most people cannot identify what you are going through. This calm and peaceful state is found in those oblivious people who are often clueless of what is going on around them. I envy these people as much as I am annoyed by them. Anyway, for whatever reason, we tend to be much more aware of what goes on around us, and we also tend to overanalyze and overthink situations. Unfortunately, that is a big part of why we are vulnerable to panic attacks.

If you have experienced panic attacks, you know they are terrorizing. It's absolutely horrible. You feel like you're going to die. You feel like, if you don't hold on very tight, everything is just going to go to pieces. Physical pain is one thing, but mental pain is so much more severe. At this point, I want to make sure that you know that I have experienced lengthy and severe panic attacks. People are different, but typically, an attack can peak in 10 to 20 to 30 min. However, you can experience ongoing attacks that never seem to end for upwards of an hour. They may even repeat themselves in a 24-hour day. As we all experience different levels of panic attacks, consider this information as a guideline.

I also want to make sure that you know that I have found my freedom from them. When I was embedded in my panic attacks, freedom and a normal life were nowhere to be found. I basically reached the point of hopelessness. However, I received my deliverance and my freedom, and you will also. I'm just reinforcing that I have probably already experienced everything that you're feeling. I'm telling you this because I want you to start opening yourself up to beginning to believe that you also will receive your freedom.

So, you experience a panic attack. The fear, the terror, the pain are debilitating. Now you develop a fear of anything that could possibly trigger another panic attack. You begin to fear "fear" itself.

Remember, when fear is based on speculation, it is based on something that can't be identified. If fear is based on what cannot be identified, then freedom from fear is not obtainable.

Panic attacks are caused by a fear that cannot be understood or identified.

However, because a fear is perceived, most of the time by the subconscious, these feelings of fear somehow have the ability to cause adrenaline to be released.

This is something the mind is not completely conscious of. Without the ability to identify a danger, the mind will not have the ability to understand what is going on. When adrenaline is released, your heart rate increases dramatically, and surges of energy go through your body.

Without any apparent danger to correlate the feelings to, the mind becomes confused. With alarming physical reactions to adrenaline, with no apparent danger, your mind enters a conclusion that you are having a physical malfunction. It is rarely a minor malfunction that the mind perceives; it most often perceives malfunctions that have the potential to result in death, such as heart attacks and strokes. Because of the confusion over the feelings that your body is experiencing, the mind now concludes that a physical malfunction is the danger, so with that conclusion, a second wave of adrenaline is released into the body. With this second wave of adrenaline, along with a tendency to be in nerve sensitization, all the feelings of a physical malfunction that triggered the second wave of adrenaline now escalates into a state of terror. Because speculation started the process, the mind is not left with concrete evidence in its attempt to logically stop that which was initiated illogically and fueled by speculation.

At this point, the best thing for me to do is to share an experience that I went through so that, hopefully, you begin to see the process of how panic attacks work and possibly even identify with what I was going through.

I'm going to share with you something that I went through at the very beginning of dealing with panic attacks, before I knew the information that I'm sharing with you in this book. Let's look back at the time I was in the grocery store. It may be easier for you to understand this time.

Deeper analysis of when I first started to experience PANIC ATTACKS

Monday was my day off work, so that was the day I always ran errands and bought groceries. I never felt uncomfortable buying groceries in the past. I grabbed my cart, made sure that I picked the one that had the least number of wheels that did not work and wasn't lopsided because there was a wad of gum attached to it, and headed on my way. About halfway through my shopping, for some reason, I experienced some unusual and bizarre feelings. I soon began to feel extremely uncomfortable. I was confused because there was no apparent reason for these feelings. There was no logical explanation. My mind could not identify any apparent danger. For some reason, subconscious thoughts perceived an imminent danger, and my body started responding to that danger. Because of the deception that I was in danger, adrenaline started being released into my bloodstream to prepare me to respond to the danger. However, the problem was that there was no danger to respond to. What was taking place caused confusion in my mind, which began to race with speculation. Speculation runs rampant when there are no concrete explanations. So, the perception of my subconscious initiated fear, which initiated the release of more adrenaline. The release of adrenaline caused my body to behave as if there was a physical malfunction. My heart was racing, it was hard to breathe, and I began to get dizzy. Now my mind had something concrete to identify as the source of fear—the perception that there was a physical malfunction. This gave my mind something concrete to fear, and more adrenaline was released into my body, which intensified the original deceptive feelings.

Going over the process again from a different angle. I was, in fact, in a safe place. For some reason, subconsciously I perceived danger that was not apparent to my mind. The subconscious perception was strong enough to trigger the release of adrenaline. I was in fear, and I was reacting to fear, but my mind was not able to identify the fear. The initial release of adrenaline caused the feeling of physical malfunctions. When my mind perceived these malfunctions without any apparent danger, speculation of physical malfunctions transferred from my subconscious to my conscious. My mind now perceived danger because of the way my body was responding to the first release of adrenaline. Continued releases of adrenaline were initiated because my mind perceived dangerous physical malfunctions.

One more time. Something in my subconscious perceived a fear that was not perceived by my mind. The perceived fear in my subconscious began to trigger adrenaline. Because my mind could not identify any apparent fear, there was no real need for this adrenaline. However, because the adrenaline was present for no reason, the reaction of the body to adrenaline was perceived as a malfunction of the body. Now that the mind perceived this malfunction, more adrenaline was released because the mind entered into speculation that what was being felt in the body was a physical malfunction severe enough that it could possibly lead to death.

By intentionally repeating the story with just subtle variations, I hope you can begin to grasp from my experiences what is going on within you to cause the way you feel.

Please understand that I am not saying that every panic or anxiety attack happens this way. However, my experience has shown me that certain obvious patterns begin to emerge that, when understood, give us the tools we need to disrupt the process before a harmless incident progresses into a full-blown panic attack.

Now that we've spent ample time in the attempt to understand what happens during a panic attack, we are prepared to set up more defenses in efforts to stop one before it has the opportunity to gain momentum to cause uncontrollable terror.

RUTS IN YOUR MIND

CAUSED BY HARMFUL THOUGHT PATTERNS

We have spent quite a bit of time learning about panic attacks. Now we are going to use what we have learned to disrupt the process in order to begin to make panic attacks ineffective. Let's review the three crucial definitions.

The definition of *fear* is "an unpleasant emotion caused by the belief that someone or something is dangerous, likely to cause pain, or become a threat."

The definition of *anxiety* is "a feeling of worry, nervousness, or unease, typically about an imminent event or something with an uncertain outcome."

The definition of *speculation* is "the forming of a theory or conjecture without firm evidence."

Through speculation, we conclude that something is a threat to us. Because we perceive a threat, the normal response is to feel fear. The problem is that we feel fear, but we cannot identify what is causing us to feel that way. Because of the confusion, anxiety will set in, which is an excellent condition for panic attacks to manifest and escalate.

When you perceive that you are in danger but cannot identify the danger, you must enter speculation. Without firm evidence, speculations can continue at a relentless pace. This keeps the fire fueled.

Unknown threat ⟶ Fear ⟶ Speculation ⟶ Confusion ⟶ Anxiety ⟶ Panic

In earlier chapters, I stated that all panic attacks are based on fear. Now we're going to take that one step further. Panic attacks are based on a fear that has escalated through speculation. Because speculations form conclusions without facts, they can be very deceiving. In that state of deception, incorrect patterns of thinking begin to emerge.

> **In the absence of truth, a lie, by default, will become your truth.**

THE LOGGING TRAIL

When in the mountains, we would drive on logging trails that were not maintained for public access. You would need a four-wheel-drive vehicle, and you would need the necessary equipment to be able to dig yourself out if your vehicle got stuck.

As vehicles continue to travel these logging trails, ruts in the trails would begin to form and would grow deeper and deeper each time a vehicle traveled that route. The ruts in the trail would soon become so deep that you did not have any choice but to follow the path that was laid out for you. Because the trail was traveled over and over and over, the ruts would become so deep that a vehicle was incapable of navigating out of the ruts.

This is crucially important to understand because this is what happens with your mind—thoughts are the vehicles; the mind is the logging trail. When thoughts are allowed to travel the same path over and over, patterns begin to emerge. The patterns are the ruts. When patterns of thinking are allowed to develop, the patterns become so embedded and familiar that the patterns of thinking become what we refer to as strongholds.

Strongholds are patterns of thinking that have taken you hostage, and to think a different way is virtually impossible.

> **Panic disorder and anxiety disorder have the ability to hold us hostage by the formation of thinking patterns that have been established by continually experiencing fear and despair.**

In the mountains, when we would drive the logging trails, we were held hostage by the ruts since the vehicle could not simply turn out of them; the ruts were too deep. If we desired to turn out of them, what we had to do was to fill in the ruts with rocks and whatever else we could find, and then we would lay a board so it became a ramp that the vehicle could drive up on so that we could navigate out of the ruts.

When dealing with the mind, we must be aware that our thoughts have been traveling the same paths for so long that patterns have been established. With panic attacks, a person has allowed incorrect or harmful thoughts to follow the same path over and over until a pattern has been developed, and eventually, a stronghold has been established. Like the vehicle, you can't just suddenly start thinking differently; you must fill in the ruts—the patterns of thoughts—with facts, with truth. As an act of your will, as an act of your own determination, together we will learn how to take incorrect thoughts captive and prevent them from continuing to run rampant and establish harmful patterns of thinking. We're going to learn how to fill in the ruts of our mind with truth so that we will begin to train our mind how to think differently.

This is so important to understand that I'm going to give you one more illustration. I often like to refer to patterns of thinking as being a runaway mind. Because your mind is continuously driven by the same pattern of thinking, a "mindset" becomes established. We will learn more about "mindset" in future chapters. What you must understand is that an incorrect pattern of thinking will eventually create an incorrect pattern of behavior. Panic and anxiety disorders cause us to develop a behavior that we want to be free from.

> The improper and unnecessary release of adrenaline plays a huge factor in panic attacks. However, even more important is understanding how to take authority over your thoughts so you are no longer held hostage to an undesirable behavior.

Look at the following example:

TRUCKS WITH NO BRAKES

A runaway *thought pattern* is like several trucks parked at the top of a very steep hill. Each truck is pointed toward a path that has been established by vehicles continually traveling the same course. Each truck is devoid of any brakes. Each truck is teetering right on the edge of the steep hill.

Let's say that the runaway thought pattern that we are dealing with is that of being an alcoholic. (As well as counseling people who suffer from panic attacks, I also counsel people who struggle with addiction, such as alcohol. Alcohol can be physically and psychologically addictive.)

So, with a person who is addicted to alcohol, their body wants alcohol. The mind has been trained by the thought pattern that to be without alcohol is not an option. Any time a person who is addicted to alcohol attempts to modify their behavior, fear gives a little nudge, just as if you were to nudge a truck teetering at the top of the hill, pushing it over the edge and plunging it into inevitable destruction. The truck represents a thought, while the hill and path represent a trained pattern of thinking. Even if a person was determined to try to change, they would not be able to, because there has been nothing done to change their runaway thoughts.

Their thoughts have been traveling the same path for so long that a pattern has been established from which there is no escape.

A course of action—without focusing on the alcohol. If the alcoholic person would start intentionally and persistently entertaining the thought that there is life outside of alcohol, they would begin to disrupt the addictive patterns of thinking. Before long, brakes would slowly be added to the trucks, and after that, cutoffs on the path would soon be established. Before long, the trucks would be moved farther back from the edge of the hill so it would take a lot more to start the runaway thought pattern.

Please understand that I know how addicting alcohol can be because I deal with it firsthand with the people that I counsel. I'm just giving you an illustration that may be oversimplified, but I believe it will help you understand what you're going through.

A person who suffers from panic attacks deals a lot with the same process. Fear has been allowed to create patterns of thinking that always find the same destination—the fear of death or the fear of a lack of control. For example, a person stubs their toe. "Ouch, that hurts!" they may exclaim. Now, for a person without a runaway thought pattern, the story would end there, but not for a person who suffers from anxiety and panic attacks. Their thought pattern would most likely be: "I'm going to lose that nail. That toe might get infected. I could lose that toe, or I could get blood poisoning and lose my foot. It could be so bad that I lose my leg. I saw on the news where a person got a blood clot from an injury and it flowed to the brain. They had a stroke and eventually died."

This sounds so absurd, but people actually think this way.

Now let's review what we learned in the last chapter to understand the process of how a panic attack occurs.

RUNAWAY
THOUGHTS

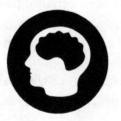

THOUGHT
PATTERNS

MINDSET

SUBCONSCIOUS

Something in my subconscious perceived fear that was not perceived by my mind. The perceived fear in my subconscious began to trigger adrenaline. My mind could not identify any apparent fear, but adrenalin was still released, even though there was no need for it. Because adrenaline was present for no reason, the reaction of the body to adrenaline was perceived as a malfunction of the body. Now that the mind perceived what was viewed as malfunctions of the body, more adrenaline was now released because the mind entered into speculation that what was being felt in the body was a physical malfunction severe enough that it could possibly lead to death.

**THE PROBLEM WITH PANIC ATTACKS IS THAT
THEY ARE COMPLETELY ILLOGICAL**

Because of your panic attack:

- You cannot intellectually comprehend what is happening.
- A fear quickly surfaces that you are having a mental breakdown or a major physical malfunction.
- Fear continues to escalate.
- Speculation runs rampant.
- You overthink everything.
- Your mind continually seeks answers that are not there.
- You live in speculation.

The result is that harmful patterns of thinking have been formed. Therefore:

- Your mind is taken hostage.
- The mindset that has been established as the result of continuous harmful thoughts no longer has the ability to control these harmful thought patterns.

When in the guts of a panic attack, my mind became so damaged by the formation of incorrect patterns of thinking that I was incapable of finding a way of escape. Rarely did a day go by that I did not entertain the thought that I could face death at any moment. This created a vicious cycle. Speculation creates fear, which causes adrenaline to be released, making you extremely uncomfortable. This causes more speculation, which, in turn, causes more fear, which releases more adrenaline.

Okay, I believe that I have covered the necessary information for you to understand how a panic attack operates. Those who deal with panic attacks will be nodding in agreement. As you share this information—this book—with your family and friends, they should be starting to grasp what you have been going through. We need this information because now we are ready to provide tangible actions to obtain a behavior modification to bring about your freedom.

LOGICALLY DEALING WITH THE ILLOGICAL

LET'S LIST WHAT WE ARE EXPERIENCING THAT IS ILLOGICAL

- I experience fear when there is no apparent danger.
- I experience symptoms in my body that are so extreme that I conclude I must be having a major physical malfunction.
- I experience fear that I find I am not able to control.
- For no apparent reason, I will suddenly feel my heart racing, find it hard to breathe, feel my chest tightening, feel tingling through my body, feel lightheaded, dizzy, and like I'm going to pass out. I often experience heart palpitations.
- I find it impossible to have fun like I once was able to.
- There are certain places that I consistently find uncomfortable.
- I find that, because of fear, I don't want to leave my house.
- I find I am always nervous and tense because I live in fear of experiencing another panic attack.
- Many times, I feel so bad that I am tempted to be taken to the emergency room because I am convinced something horrible is wrong with my health.

Because of all the information provided in the last few chapters, I believe you are gaining insight into what is causing the problem. Now we're going to logically identify the problems, and we're going to logically embrace the solutions.

The following are reasons for experiencing panic attacks in your life. You may find that there is one main reason, or you may find that it is a combination of reasons. Don't worry, we will find a way out of this mess.

REASONS FOR PANIC ATTACKS

YOU

- Are oversensitive to adrenaline.
- Can't control the way you think.
- Can't change the way you think.
- Have developed harmful patterns of thinking.
- Have a tendency to overthink things and overanalyze things.
- Have a constant fear of death.

AND

Your subconscious perceives a fear that is not evident to your mind.

As we discuss the solutions, again, I'm going to assume that your panic attacks are severe to debilitating. I'm going to start with solutions that will immediately slow down panic attacks and we will continue to adopt solutions until you are finally free from this nightmare.

#1- Get a physical

If you have not done this yet, I'm encouraging you as strongly as I can to take the time to do it. Get as much medical attention as you need to enable you to walk away convinced that you are in good health.

The reason – *Panic attacks are fueled by speculation and fear.*

The definition of *speculation* is "the forming of a theory or conjecture without firm evidence."

The *definition* of fear is "an unpleasant emotion caused by the belief that someone or something is dangerous, likely to either cause pain or become a threat."

We're going to start by removing potential fuel from the fire. Until we get things firmly under control, adrenaline is going to cause you to feel like something is physically wrong with your body. Therefore, I need you to be prepared to resist speculation. I need you to be very strong to resist entering into fear.

For whatever reason, excess adrenaline will most likely be released in your body. There will be no logical explanation for the way you feel because there will not be any identifiable danger.

As soon as you feel the effects of adrenaline on your body and experience the uncomfortable side effects, I need you to be convinced that you are not in a life-threatening situation. You had a physical. Even though you feel horrible, we know that adrenaline is a reason for the way you feel. I need you to learn how to resist fear.

The process will go something like this. You will be somewhere when suddenly you will feel the effects of adrenaline being released into your bloodstream. You will feel all the symptoms that we have gone over and over. I need you to logically accept that there is no danger, but that, for some reason, adrenaline was released. I need you to disregard the way you feel instead of allowing speculation to take you to a place of fear. When you feel the onset of the effects of adrenaline, I need you to speak out loud and with much conviction.

It will go something like this:

"I feel horrible. I feel horrible because adrenaline has just been released into my body for no apparent reason. Even though I feel horrible, I am not in any danger. I just had a complete physical, and every organ

and every tissue of my body functions perfectly. I refuse to enter into fear because there is nothing to fear. I refuse to speculate. There is nothing wrong. I can deal with the way I feel because the effects of the adrenaline will pass quickly."

If done correctly, you will begin to feel the fear begin to dissipate and the effects of the adrenaline will begin to leave your body. This is the way to gain back control.

In just a little while, I will explain why it's so important to speak out loud. For now, I just need you to trust me. This sounds so simple, but you will find that doing this will begin to reduce the fear and anxiety.

> By speaking words that we choose to believe, that go against the way we feel, we are beginning to learn the process of disrupting harmful thought patterns. We are also beginning the process of creating a new "mindset."

What I'm telling you to do has to be done immediately at the onset of fear or panic. You must speak in complete opposition to any thoughts of fear and speculation of danger. If you have to, take some notecards and write out your declarations of faith. Put them on the notepad of your smartphone. Do whatever you have to in order to be prepared to speak against what you are feeling.

The reason that you obtained a complete physical is so that you can logically put to rest any illogical conclusions that your mind has been conditioned to accept through speculation. The reason that you speak in opposition to the way your mind has been trained to think is that the way your mind has been trained is the result of continually entertaining harmful negative thoughts. Again, what we are learning to do is to disrupt harmful thought patterns.

The reason that I want you to get a physical is so that you have firm evidence that your health is sound. Firm evidence is what you need to put an end to harmful speculation.

#2 – Medication

Initially, I found it necessary to take medication to help me overcome panic attacks. Medication is important, but I would say that the information that we are learning is just as, if not more, important.

Too often, I have seen people who rely solely on medication to get their panic attacks under control but who do not receive freedom from continually experiencing the attacks.

As said before, I often compare medications to a cast on a broken leg. To simplify things, we could basically say that your mind is "broken." No, you're not insane or mentally ill; your mind has been beaten up and bruised by experiencing continued panic attacks.

My suggestion is that, along with your physical, you begin to take medication as prescribed and if deemed necessary by your physician. Remember, I am not a licensed physician. The direction and suggestions from your doctor must always supersede what I tell you. The information that I am giving you is based on my own experiences and those people that I counsel with.

Medications often come with some scary side effects. However, your doctor should be able to walk you through what is believed to be the best. Pharmacists are also a good resource. Some of the medications used fall into different categories. Your doctor may decide that medication should be part of your therapy to lessen your attacks' physical symptoms. It might be part of the first step in your road to freedom. For instance, your doctor might prescribe you antidepressants, anti-anxiety meds or medications to even out an irregular heartbeat or heart palpitations, and meds to treat high blood pressure, if needed.

Medication helped me in my early stages of dealing with panic attacks. Again, you must rely on the opinion and the direction of your doctor.

If you are having severe to debilitating panic attacks, medication will be very helpful in your initial effort to begin to reduce the frequency and the severity of the attacks. Please rely on your doctor's opinion. My help will be a blessing in the non-medical aspects of dealing with panic attacks.

#3- Capturing and rerouting thoughts

What I'm going to teach you now is what I found to be the most helpful to obtaining my freedom from panic attacks. We are going to cover this topic in depth in the next few chapters.

Doctors and medications are extremely helpful, but if you plan on obtaining your freedom as opposed to just maintaining control of your panic attacks, you're probably going to have to take the course of action that I did.

My panic attacks had a debilitating control over me; however, I knew I wasn't going to live the rest of my life like that. Here was my course of action:

- I had to learn to change the way I think.
- I had to reconstruct thought patterns.
- I had to take irrational thoughts captive.
- I had to learn to identify speculation and put a stop to it.
- I had to learn to stop overanalyzing everything.
- I had to learn how to stop harmful runaway thoughts.
- I had to develop a new mindset.
- I had to enlist the help of some good friends.

The first thing I wanted you to know was a difference between an "anxiety attack" versus a "panic attack."

You see, initially, a lot of people kept telling me that what I was going through was just a reaction to stress. However, I knew it wasn't merely stress-related. Stress may play a part, but it is not the whole story. This is important for you to know:

In an *anxiety attack*, people may feel fearful, apprehensive, or nervous, have a racing heart, tight chest, or be short of breath (these are some of the symptoms they have in common). In many cases, it can be short-lived. When the stressor goes away, so does the anxiety attack. Anxiety attacks are generally less intense and based on the persistent worry of usually known stressors. They can come on slower and may be persistent and long-lasting if the object of the worry is a stronghold in your way of thinking. Unlike a panic attack, the symptoms of anxiety may be persistent and very long-lasting—days, weeks, or even months if deep ruts have become rooted in your mindset, and the stressors remain. This is more prevalent when it co-exists with depression.

With a *panic attack*, you may feel anxiety, but the panic attack doesn't come in reaction to a stressor. It's unprovoked, and it's unpredictable. The result is sheer terror, its intensity far greater than that of an anxiety attack. Although some panic attacks can peak within 10 dreadful minutes, they can crop up in succession. When this happens, it is difficult to know when one ends and another begins.

A lot of people have written a lot of things about panic and anxiety attacks. I've gained some insight from what has been written, but most of what I'm teaching you is derived from first-hand experience.

I'm going to mostly refer to panic attacks because I feel like your ability to overcome panic attacks will also give you the ability to overcome any anxiety attack.

The basis of a panic attack is fear. I do not know all the scientific and medical information of what is happening, but I do understand how my mind works, I do understand why I feel the way I do, and I do understand how to gain control over fear.

Because we're dealing with fear, I'm going to teach you how to disrupt it and get it under control. I've had a lot of hands-on experience with counseling people, which has helped me understand what works and what doesn't work. Ultimately, I rely on the Word of God because I know that God made me and I can use the wisdom of God to learn how to correct what is broken.

Okay, we've covered medical help, and we have covered the importance of medication. Now we are going to begin to learn applications that will ultimately free you up from panic attacks.

Since the basis of a panic attack is fear, we're going to learn how to take away the source of fear—speculation.

Remember, we are dealing with a combination of the following factors:

- The release of adrenaline when there is no identifiable danger.
- Confusion as to why you feel the effects of adrenaline when there is no identifiable danger.
- Thoughts have traveled the same negative path for so long that patterns of negative, damaging thinking have been established and it's hard to think differently.
- The tendency to overthink and overanalyze.
- The tendency to worry way too much.

I believe anxiety attacks are different than panic attacks in that, with an anxiety attack, you can identify the source of the anxiety that you are experiencing and conclude that the level of anxiety that you face is just too much for you to handle.

Panic attacks may happen in different ways with different causes, but I'm going to start with what I feel is most common. We've gone over this before, so I'll just briefly recap so that I can lay out our line of attack to obtain freedom.

> <u>The most common form of panic attack:</u> for some reason, fear causes a release of adrenaline into my body. The fear initiates from my subconscious because my mind is not aware of any danger. Somehow adrenaline is released for no apparent reason. The body reacts to the adrenaline, which is very scary when you don't identify anything that would seem dangerous. When adrenaline is released, the body overreacts with wild symptoms. The mind now releases a second wave of adrenaline because of the fear initiated from how the body reacted to the first release of adrenaline. Though you are in a non-threatening situation, you are in total fear. As adrenaline keeps flowing into your bloodstream, the symptoms worsen until you become convinced you're probably going to die.

I often refer to adrenaline being dispensed into your bloodstream in levels, but I'm sure that adrenaline can also just be a constant flow that becomes way too much for the person to handle because of the extreme effects that are felt in their body.

Now, the solution. Forgive me for repeating myself so often, but the more you understand and internalize this information, the more it becomes the foundation of your arsenal for defense and readily retrievable to pull from your long-term memory in times of need. The more you understand what is going on, the more effective you will be at using the solution tactics.

FEAR, THOUGHTS, BEHAVIOR

The way you think is ultimately going to control the way you behave. We need a behavioral change, so we will start by controlling the way we think. Believe me, this is not that "mind over matter" teaching—this is tangible and effective.

I want you to do something. You will need to get someone to help you. You're going to count from 1 to 20 in your mind. Instruct the person helping you to tell you to say something out loud, like your name, while you are silently counting. While counting in your mind, to yourself, say something out loud. Many people find that their counting stops after doing this.

This is absolutely huge. The way we are going to fight panic attacks is to disrupt the harmful thought patterns we create. Harmful thought patterns have been established by constantly thinking the same way. Any time thoughts get anywhere near the pattern that has been established, your mind will go right to that same conclusion.

I mentioned this process when we were talking about initially seeking medical help. Now we're going to take this process and really put it to work.

PROTECT YOUR EARS AND EYES

To change our behavior, we're going to change the way we think, so we are going to have to be very selective in what we allow ourselves to hear and see.

Have you ever gotten a song in your head and then go all day trying to get it out of your head? Of course you have. The thing that we have to be so watchful of is that we never allow anything we see or hear to get into our head that can fuel the fire of speculation. Again, I'm not dealing with oblivious people. Most people who deal with panic attacks are sharp and attentive. We are simply people who think too much and speculate about the wrong things.

STOP

> Stop watching movies and TV programs that deal with excessive drama and horror. Stop watching those crazy medical programs where somebody is always being diagnosed with something that is fatal.
>
> Stop listening to music that is negative. Remove yourself from situations where people are complaining and sharing their tales of woe.
>
> Do not entertain any activity involving fear or horror.

I don't know about you, but every time that I was around someone who had a very serious physical ailment and would share all the gory details of it with me, I found myself adopting the same symptoms. Why? Two reasons. First, as a victim of panic attacks, I would overthink and overanalyze. Second, my thoughts were trained to be based on fear and self-preservation.

To stop watching certain movies and TV programs may sound drastic, but you must decide just how much you want to be free from what you're experiencing.

For myself, when I first began to understand how panic attacks worked, I would restrict myself to only watching good, clean comedy TV. Along with that, I restricted what I listened to. I would get recordings of the promises of God and would constantly have them playing into my ear. I had to remove any potentially harmful speculation, and I had to change the way I thought by changing what I was constantly exposed to.

TAKE THOUGHTS CAPTIVE

I came to understand that, for me, panic attacks would be triggered by two main avenues.

First, subconsciously I would fear something in my mind that I could not identify. Adrenaline would be released into my body, and I became extremely hyper and nervous, with a racing heart and difficulty breathing. Because my mind could not identify any danger, fear would develop with the speculation that I was having a major physical crisis, and more adrenaline would be released, which catapulted the initial symptoms and feelings into a potential meltdown.

Second, I developed a fear of fear. I dreaded the prospect of a panic attack, so much so that I became so watchful over any little symptom that made me think that I was potentially being set up to experience another one.

Panic attacks can occur differently than what I've just described, but ultimately, the solution for becoming free will be the same no matter what initiates the attack.

> **Learn to take thoughts captive. The first thing that I instructed you to do was to minimize potential speculation by being very selective in what you hear and what you see. Now that we have begun to start reducing negative thoughts, we want to learn how to take thoughts captive.**

In my deliverance from panic attacks, learning these first two steps gave me my first ray of hope.

When I first started to experience panic attacks, I was really getting beaten up. I started to realize that my thoughts were very negative and out of control. What I learned to do was to use the process that I taught you when I asked you to count to 20 and then have someone ask you a question.

What I learned was that, if I wanted to stop the way I was thinking, I had to do it by speaking out the opposite of the way I was feeling.

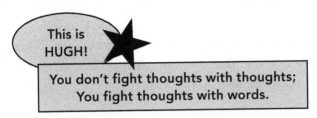

This is HUGH!

You don't fight thoughts with thoughts;
You fight thoughts with words.

The way I took negative thoughts captive was to speak aloud things that were contrary to those negative thoughts. Any time a negative thought would surface, I would capture that thought by disputing it with words of truth and faith.

When, for some reason, your subconscious perceives a fear that is not identifiable by your mind, adrenaline is released, and your mind starts racing with thoughts of why your body is reacting the way it does. Knowing that, I found that as soon as I began to feel the release of adrenaline, I would be all primed to start speaking words that would have the ability to disrupt the thoughts that, up to this time, had been allowed to run rampant.

Panic attacks are fueled by fear. Fear is fueled by speculation. Speculation creates harmful negative thoughts. Stop the negative thoughts, and harmful speculation will begin to fizzle out. Remove the fuel for fear, and you will remove the fuel for panic attacks.

If you understand this, you're now on the correct path that leads to freedom.

DEVELOP NEW PATTERNS OF THINKING

I want you to learn how to effectively capture thoughts and then to develop new patterns of thinking.

I first reduced the negative information that my mind was exposed to. Taking thoughts captive and developing new patterns of thinking go hand in hand. It might be good for you to go back and review the section that we covered about the ruts in the logging trails. If you remember, we had to fill in the ruts if we wanted to get the vehicle to move in a different direction. In the same way, your mind develops patterns of thinking. Therefore, we first must capture the incorrect thoughts by speaking words that oppose the negative speculation.

I spent time writing down the way I wanted to believe as opposed to the harmful patterns that were already established in my mind. I would speak against any harmful feeling and would constantly make statements of faith out loud.

Just a quick recap on our practical application:

1. Get a complete and thorough physical.
2. Begin medication when necessary under the direction of your physician.
3. Protect your ears and eyes.
4. Capture and reroute your thoughts to develop a new mindset.

CONTROL THE WAY YOU THINK IN ORDER TO CONTROL THE WAY YOU BEHAVE.

TAKING BACK CONTROL
OF YOUR MIND

What I'm going to teach you is so effective that it will not only bring freedom from panic attacks, but it will also offer help for those who deal with:

- Debilitating anxiety
- Excessive and abnormal stress
- Depression
- Excessive nervousness
- Uncontrolled thoughts
- Certain addictions
- Those whose lives are devoid of peace, joy, and contentment

The reason that I've spent so much time educating you about panic attacks is that you're going to find that information vital for what we're going to achieve to obtain your freedom. Even if you do not suffer from panic attacks specifically, but rather find that you struggle with any excessive fear or mental torment, and these have affected your behavior (i.e., *the way you live life), then* read about what I'm going to teach very carefully. Get ready to be transformed.

Your success will be completely dependent on just how desperate you are to obtain your freedom. From this point on, I need you to be determined, relentless, and aggressive, and you can even mix in a portion of anger. Something has robbed you of the quality of your life, and that something must be exposed. We must put an end to it.

To obtain your freedom, I'm going to teach you about:

- Mental barriers
- Thought boundaries
- Mindsets

We are going to learn about them and put them into practice immediately.

The reason I am so insistent on you seeing a doctor and getting a complete and thorough physical exam is so that we can begin the process of putting boundaries on your thoughts.

Panic attacks can cause a person to entertain thoughts that someone else would never entertain.

People often ask me if I still experienced panic attacks. I tell them, no, because I have learned to control the way I think. Do I have the potential to have panic attacks? Absolutely. However, I have established limits on and strict guidelines for any thoughts that I now entertain.

I may feel uncomfortable at times, but I will not allow speculation to drive me to have thoughts about catastrophic outcomes. I do not allow myself to entertain thoughts of heart attacks, strokes, or any other potentially life-threatening occurrences. Why? Because I have put a boundary on my thoughts. Any thoughts that try to operate outside that boundary, I take captive, and I reroute them.

Over the years, I have counseled many people who suffer from panic attacks. A lot of them have my phone number and a lot of people know and feel comfortable that they can call me 24/7.

MAGGIE'S STORY

One night, or should I say one morning, at about 2 a.m., I received a frantic call from a friend of mine, Maggie. She was calling me to tell me that she was going to call the ambulance to take her to the emergency room.

"Why?" I asked.

"Because I am dying. My heart is racing, I can't breathe, I have pain in my chest, and I feel tingling in my hands and my feet. Also, I think my lips are numb," she replied.

I then told Maggie, "Before you call the ambulance, let me ask you a few important questions. Who should I contact? Should I come over to the house to make sure things are shut, turned off, and locked up?"

My game plan was to cause her to think about something other than the way she felt. *I had to help her disrupt her harmful pattern of thinking*; in other words, I had to re-direct her thought pattern. She did not know what I was up to, so she became engaged in my questioning.

After I had her attention, I asked her a wild question. "You have a really cool dog, I really like that dog; it's such a good pet. If you die, do you mind if I keep the dog for myself?"

Her response was a mixture of anger and confusion. "What are you talking about? Why would you ask me something as stupid as that?"

"Well," I said, "it sounds most likely that you're going to die from whatever you are experiencing, so if I don't get to talk to you again, I just want to make sure that I get to keep your dog."

Along with her initial anger, she hurled a few graphic words at me (words that would be inappropriate to mention in a book like this). Then I made a statement: "By the way, your breathing sounds better."

There was a moment of silence before she remarked, "My breathing is better. My heart is not beating as fast as it was."

Then I said, "Oh no, does this mean you're not going to die? I really had my hopes set on adopting your dog!"

She finally caught on to what I was doing, and she started laughing. All those horrible symptoms left her, and I continued to joke with her about anything that I could come up with that would make her laugh.

So, what happened here?

I disrupted her thought patterns long enough for her to receive some relief from the horrible symptoms that she was experiencing.

When I am helping people get through a panic attack, I first attempt to get their attention, so they take their eyes off themselves. Then I try to get them laughing about something—anything. Over the years, I have discovered that laughter is a very effective tool for slowing down and even stopping the flow of adrenaline into your body.

Unfortunately, thoughts of fear initiate the release of adrenaline. If a fear stems from actual danger, the adrenaline is welcomed because the adrenaline will help you deal with the danger. If the fear stems from merely a perceived danger, then the adrenaline is unwelcome because there is no need for it.

The important thing to realize is that the body cannot discern between a real and a perceived danger. We were created in a way that the body releases adrenaline based on our thoughts. The body does not sit down with the mind to discuss whether you are truly in danger or whether, for some reason, your subconscious perceives a danger that isn't really there. The body doesn't sit down with the mind and do lunch or enjoy a time of coffee and dialogue. No, your body is designed to react to your mind—to the thoughts based on the conclusion of the perception. We will discuss this later in greater depth, but it is vital that you understand the relationship between the reaction of the body and the thoughts of the mind.

Anyway, regarding Maggie's situation, any time that I can get someone laughing, I find that the release of adrenaline and some of the drastic feelings of adrenaline in the body will dissipate.

I disrupted her thought pattern to the extent that she no longer perceived danger, so her mind no longer initiated any further releases of adrenaline.

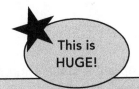

This is HUGE!

If you perceive danger, laughter will not be the outcome. If we engage in the outcome of laughter, we disrupt the pattern of harmful perception.

If you are laughing, your mind must come to the conclusion that you are no longer in danger. If the mind perceives that there is no danger, there will be no demand placed on the body to release adrenaline. When the adrenaline stops, the alarming symptoms in the body stop, so the racing of the mind with thoughts based on speculation finally comes to an end.

By the way, *Proverbs 17:22* the Word of God makes mention of this. Laughter is awesome. Laughter is like a body massage for the inside of you!

I'm going to teach you more about the effectiveness of laughter as soon as I make it clear why it has the ability to be so effective. Also, I'm going to refer back to this story with Maggie to help you better understand how to put the upcoming principles to work.

First up, we're going to learn about *mental barriers.*

I want to give you an example of just how strong of an influence *a mental barrier* can have on a person's behavior.

THE GOOD AND THE BAD OF A MENTAL BARRIER

> **A mental barrier can stand in the way of something awesome that someone would like to achieve. It can also be used to begin taking harmful thoughts captive in order to disrupt destructive thought patterns.**

THE 4-MINUTE MILE

In track and field, there was a belief that it was impossible to run a mile in less than four minutes. Therefore, a mental barrier had been established in the minds of people. However, on May 6, 1954, Roger Bannister was the first man on record to prove that belief to be wrong.

History shows that runners had chased the dream of breaking the four-minute mile since 1886. During all those years, no one was able to run a four-minute mile until Roger did in 1954. Amazingly, less than two months later, on June 21, 1954, John Landy broke the four-minute mile and did it in a faster time than Roger Bannister.

Now, a little over a half a century later, thousands of runners have conquered the four-minute mile. Why? Because one runner broke the barrier that other runners were being held hostage to. Hence, it is important to note that the way a person thinks will determine the way they behave. When everyone viewed the four-minute mile as impossible, their behavior lined up with the mental barrier. When the barrier was destroyed, people's thoughts were no longer held captive, so their behavior was no longer restricted.

When barriers were established and runners accepted those established barriers, the runners could not change their behavior because their thoughts determined their behavior.

So, what in the world is my point with all this? I want you to understand the strength of mental barriers, and I want you to learn to use them for your deliverance.

In the case of the four-minute mile, the mental barrier that was established prevented the behavior of runners from breaking the four-minute mile because they could not entertain the thought of running a mile in less than four minutes. It is crucial to understand that *the way you think is ultimately going to determine the way you behave.*

Mental barriers prevent thoughts from entertaining a possibility, whether good or bad. Since running a four-minute mile is a good thing, when the mental barrier was finally destroyed, people now could entertain thoughts that they could run faster, which, in turn, enabled them to adapt their behavior from what they thought to what they believed.

In the case of panic attacks, or any other kind of mental anxiety and torment, we have behavior that is very unfavorable. We don't want that behavior; we don't like that behavior. We don't like our behavior being controlled by fear.

Our line of attack is not to merely break down an established barrier. Our line of attack is to actually create new mental barriers that set limits (like a governor on an engine) that direct thoughts to that which we desire. Remember: to get out of the logging ruts, we had to fill the rut so that it created a type of ramp. The vehicle could no longer just travel along the well-worn ruts; it would instead, allow you to pull out of the rut and go onto the new path. Therefore, this new skill set will help you modify any behavior that we want to rid ourselves of.

People who suffer from panic attacks and anxiety disorder, for one reason or another, lack a mental barrier that is crucial in keeping fear and anxiety in a proper perspective.

The way I learned about mental barriers is that I found that my friends did not entertain the thoughts that I was prone to. Therefore, I found that my friends did not have harmful behavior patterns in reference to fear like I had.

In a lot of ways, mental barriers are the same as mental blocks; however, I like to use the term barrier because it gives me a better visual of what I'm working with.

I wrote this book in a way that it bombards you with information and situations that you can relate to. Some of the information is repetitive for a reason. I wanted to make sure that you believed that what I experienced was the same or similar to what you are experiencing. Also, as you gain more insight into the beast of panic attacks, the information will take on deeper meanings. By being an example of someone who was freed from what you're going through, my book can open up hope so that you can receive your freedom. Repetition also serves as a way of memorizing information that will be useful to call upon, even in the throes of a full-blown panic attack, as you are gaining back control of your life.

You see, panic attacks are so painful and relentless that a person begins to lose hope of ever receiving their freedom. For you, I want to be the example of the person who "broke the four-minute mile" so that you will be able to entertain thoughts that will empower you to ultimately change your behavior.

I want to destroy the mental barrier that keeps you from entertaining the thoughts of freedom. Then the way that we are going to obtain and maintain your freedom is to construct mental barriers that enable you to end harmful patterns of thinking so that we can end harmful and painful patterns of behavior.

This is going to get a little heavy, so hang in there. I will give you a lot of illustrations that will help you understand what I'm teaching. I will also give you very specific instructions as to how to apply what we have learned.

Before Roger Bannister broke the four-minute mile, there was a mental barrier that kept people from believing that it was possible. They were not able to entertain the thought that it was possible.

Once the impossible was accomplished, people were now able to entertain thoughts that enabled them to obtain a new behavior. The way you think is ultimately going to determine the way you behave.

Certain mental barriers are very healthy because they prevent harmful thinking that opens the door to harmful behavior.

> For people who suffer from panic attacks, anxiety disorders, or any other behavior that is extremely unpleasant, for one reason or another, they do not have healthy mental barriers that serve as a block from constantly entertaining extreme thoughts based on speculation.

I certainly became painfully aware that I did not possess a healthy mental barrier! Without a healthy mental barrier, thoughts of fear are allowed to run rampant, and because of that, uncontrollable fear led to harmful, unwanted behavior.

CHARLIE THE GOAT

As an illustration to help you understand this concept, I'm going to teach you about raising goats. At our restaurant and motor inn, we have a petting zoo for people to enjoy. Goats are a big attraction, and I like to raise them. They are ornery and stubborn—a lot like me. My most ornery goat was named Charlie.

Goats, like people, always seem to want what they can't have. They eat almost anything and will most likely destroy everything that is within their reach. Wow, that sounds like a lot of my friends.

So anyway, mix those two traits together, and you get a goat. Goats want what they can't have, and goats always like to be chewing on something. Because of these two traits, goats will often challenge the fence in which they are contained. Therefore, take note that the NEW barriers you build need to be higher and stronger so that even the Charlies would not be up for the challenge, and Charlie challenged everything!

Goats are herd animals, so by nature, they like to stick together somewhat. Because of that, if you ever left a goat out of the pen, that goat would most likely destroy anything that was in its path; however, it would be unlikely to run away. Most of the time, a goat on its own will return to the area that they are familiar with, back to where other goats are.

Every once in a while, you will have a goat like Charlie who is just relentless in challenging the boundaries that are established by the fence of their pen. One way or another, that goat will find a way of escape.

Since I am as ornery as a goat, I was up for the challenge of ending Charlie's escape. The motivation of the goat is to explore new territories to find new things to chew on and destroy. So, what needs to be done is to put a muzzle on the goat and then allow the goat to go through the gate and have its freedom.

With a muzzle, the goat can drink water but it cannot eat or chew on anything. I also want to make sure that the area that the goat has left to explore is devoid of anything that the goat might be likely to find enticing.

Not only do I want to keep the goat from eating, but I also want to restrict what the goat will perceive that it wants to get access to.

Once frustrated outside the pen, I allow time for the goat to eventually find its way back to the pen. Instead of letting the goat in, I feed the *other* goats on the inside of the pen while my ornery escapee, Charlie is on the outside looking in.

Aside from the regular food, I throw in some small tree branches because, for some reason, goats love gnawing on junk like that. Once my ornery wanderer has had enough of being outside the pen with *no* gratification, I take off the muzzle and put him back in the pen. The goat thoroughly enjoys the food and the "chew toys." Before long, after a few repeat performances, the former escapee begins to lose his desire for the unknown. Charlie is kinda stupid like that.

When you are training a goat, the last thing that you want is to feed it while it is outside the pen.

SCRUTINIZING MAGGIE'S STORY - WHAT CAN WE LEARN?

Okay, here are the players:

- Goats represent your thoughts.
- My ornery goat Charlie represents rampant unwanted thoughts.
- The fence represents the mind barrier.
- Food outside the fence represents feeding negative thoughts by entertaining them.
- Provisions inside the fence represent a correct mindset.

Okay, let's go back to the story of Maggie. Where did she go wrong?

Charlie (her thoughts) went AWOL and took a lot of his goat friends with him.

Maggie wasn't observant; she didn't detect the prison break. The only thing that Maggie perceived was that something was terribly wrong.

Instead of knowing what was wrong and muzzling the goats, through ignorance, she started feeding them. In other words, Maggie not only fed negative thoughts by entertaining them, but through fear, she spoke them aloud - "I am dying. My heart is racing, I can't breathe, I have pain in my chest, and I feel tingling in my hands and my feet. Also, I think my lips are numb."

We feed thoughts by continually entertaining them. We entertain them by speculation. Speculation is the forming of a thought or a belief without firm evidence.

Watch this process carefully:

✓ For whatever reason, Maggie is a person who is vulnerable to experiencing panic attacks.

- ✓ Maggie woke up in the middle the night and experienced alarming physical symptoms. Her heart was racing and pounding, she had trouble breathing, she was lightheaded, and she felt surges of energy shooting through her body.
- ✓ For one reason or another, adrenaline was released into Maggie's bloodstream. It could've been the result of a nightmare, or it could have been caused by the subconscious entertaining the presence of danger that was not apparent to her conscious mind.
- ✓ Because of the adrenaline that was released into her bloodstream, her body kicked into a fight or flight mode.
- ✓ Because she could not wrap her mind around any apparent danger, she was then forced to assume that what she was dealing with was a physical malfunction, i.e., like the onset of a heart attack or stroke.
- ✓ At that point, she had thoughts that had broken past a healthy mental barrier. In other words, the goats had gotten out of the pen and were starting to do damage.
- ✓ Instead of capturing the goats, putting muzzles on them, and guiding them back to the pen, she fed the goats that had escaped.

When you have thoughts that escape a safe mental barrier, they must be taken captive. You begin to take them captive when you refuse to yield, meditate, or speak them out loud. In other words, you don't encourage the goats by feeding them where you do not want them.

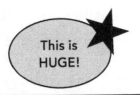

This is HUGE!

You fuel harmful negative thoughts by meditating on them, which gives them substance. When you entertain the negative harmful thoughts often enough, you create a pattern for those thoughts to follow. The reason that a person finds it is so hard to control their thoughts is that they have created a rut—a pattern for those thoughts to follow. It gets to the point where a person is incapable of thinking differently than the thought pattern or rut that is established.

The way you take thoughts captive is to

**speak out loud, speak words opposed
to the way you are thinking.**
Your mind has to stop thinking to see what your mouth has to say. The way to stop a harmful thought pattern is to do just the opposite of what Maggie did. You don't feed the thought by entertaining it, meditating on it, or talking about it. You take the thought captive by speaking words out loud that contradict the harmful thought. Over time, harmful thought patterns will eventually be filled in by truth so that thoughts will not always be held hostage to end up at the same harmful conclusion.

When you have the onset of a release of adrenaline, it is going to cause alarming physical symptoms. If you deal with the release of adrenaline properly, you can minimize the damage. If you yield to speculation, you begin to feed the harmful thoughts that have emerged.

- ✓ Maggie fed the thoughts through speculation. Speculation caused her to entertain thoughts that brought her to the conclusion that she was in a life-threatening situation.
- ✓ Because she allowed thoughts to entertain danger, the fear that she yielded to sent a message to the body to release more adrenaline.

✓ With the release of additional adrenaline, anything that Maggie felt initially was magnified significantly. Because thoughts were left outside of the mental barrier and then those thoughts were fed, things got out of hand very quickly.

This is huge. Let's review: You fuel harmful negative thoughts by meditating on them, which gives them substance. When you entertain the negative harmful thoughts often enough, you create a pattern for those thoughts to follow. The reason that a person finds it so hard to control their thoughts is that they have actually created a rut, a pattern for those thoughts to follow. It gets to the point where a person is incapable of thinking differently than the thought pattern or rut that is established. The way you take thoughts captive is to speak out loud words opposed to the way you are thinking. Your mind must stop thinking to see what your mouth has to say. The way to stop a harmful thought pattern is to do just the opposite of what Maggie did. You don't feed the thought by entertaining it, by meditating on it; you take the thought captive by speaking words out loud that contradict the harmful thought. Over time, harmful thought patterns will eventually be filled in by truth so that thoughts will not always be held hostage to end up at the same harmful conclusion

At this point, Maggie called me. So, what did I do?

Since I knew that Maggie received regular physical exams, it gave me a lot of confidence to deal with what she was going through. At this point, it was easy for me to detect that she was struggling with the effects of adrenaline and runaway thoughts. Immediately, I worked to reroute her thinking. I did this so that I could start helping her take *her* thoughts captive.

I started by asking Maggie questions that made her think about anything other than the way she was feeling. Notice that I did not simply demand that she stop thinking the thoughts she had; instead, I rerouted her attention to redirect her line of thinking. You don't have the ability to just end a thought pattern without adopting a new one.

I knew if I could stop the thoughts of fear, I could help her get to the point where her body was no longer releasing adrenaline into her bloodstream. In other words, I had to get a hold of Charlie and round up the rest of his posse and begin to do damage control. I had to remove the available food for the goats outside the pen. Specifically, I had to stop Maggie from entertaining her thoughts of fear by continually feeding into those thoughts by speculation. It was time to get rid of speculation and bring truth into the picture.

Since goats are herd animals, they will eventually return to where they are used to being. Thoughts are the same way. When you develop a safe haven for your thoughts and put up barriers, they will tend to confine themselves to where they belong; that is, within the limits of what you deem acceptable.

Once I was finally able to get Maggie laughing, her body received the message that the perceived danger was gone. At this point, the adrenaline stopped, and the effects of the adrenaline began to dissipate.

When I use the example of the goats, here are the references. Take your time to be sure you grasp the idea.

- Remember that the goats are my thoughts.
- Consider the fence as a mental barrier that I establish and am responsible for maintaining.
- Beyond the fence is a place where thoughts run wild and where thoughts do damage.
- A muzzle can control whether the goat eats or not. I put a muzzle on my thoughts by taking thoughts captive, which I do by refusing to feed them. On the other hand, I DO NOT give thoughts the ability to cause damage by entertaining them or allowing them to gain momentum through the interjection of speculation.
- *Charlie is an ornery thought that I must retrain. This is accomplished by never feeding him when he is out of line with the behavior that I desire to live with.*

- I take thoughts captive by intentionally speaking words that are in contrast to the way I feel. I must refuse to allow my feelings to determine how I think; I must purposefully choose my thoughts and words to determine how I want to feel.
- I take thoughts captive by speaking about how I desire to feel as opposed to meditating on the fickleness of my feelings. By having the ability to take my thoughts captive, I have the ability to limit the amount of adrenaline that is released into my body, and I also have the ability to limit the impact that the release of adrenaline has on my body.

ESTABLISHING THOUGHT BOUNDARIES

Now is the time to lay out the specific steps as to what I did to defeat my panic attacks, and then I'm going to lay out a very specific plan of action. Drawing information from your growing defense arsenal, we will now create a specific plan of action.

I'm a very determined person who is annoyingly relentless. Therefore, as soon as I was able to identify what was happening to me, I knew that I would find the path to freedom.

Being desperate and ornery, just like Charlie, I was not going to simply maintain a panic attack; I was going to overcome it and defeat it.

FIRST THINGS FIRST—DEVELOPING A NEW MINDSET

Have you ever been around a person who is incapable of thinking and speaking positively? How about people who always put themselves down? How about people who are consumed with self-pity? Probably sounds a lot like a family reunion. Well, anyway, there is a reason why people think and speak the way they do, and these patterns of thought are determined by their mindsets.

Mindset—a mental attitude or inclination. A fixed state of mind. The established set of attitudes held by someone that influences the development of a thought.

It has been proven scientifically that two people can be exposed to the exact same circumstances and situations but have completely different responses and completely different levels of success in dealing with what they face. The deciding factor is how a person thinks, because this is ultimately going to decide how a person behaves.

I realized that my friends could be exposed to exactly the same things that I was exposed to, only they would react in a different manner.

Somehow, over time, I developed a mindset that caused me to process information in a way that always had the ability to make me vulnerable. This evolved by entertaining too many thoughts that were associated with negative outcomes.

Living by my feelings was a downfall. It drove me to speculate way too much, which caused me to overthink and analyze everything.

To obtain my freedom, I knew that I needed to live by truth, not by feelings.

If you had a friend who lied to you as much as your feelings lie to you, you would probably no longer listen to that person, and that person would probably no longer be your friend.

My feelings would lie to me because I would allow them to. I would allow my feelings to cause me to entertain thoughts of fear, disappointment, potential failure, and even death.

WHY A NEW MINDSET IS IMPORTANT

Behavioral science documents that, on average, a person entertains about 20,000 to 50,000 thoughts a day. Yikes! That's a lot. Of course, the way I would overanalyze and overthink things, I could probably double that number. As a side note, I have some oblivious friends who would probably be hard-pressed to break 100 worthwhile, intelligent thoughts a day.

Okay, enough of my sarcasm. Not only has it been proven that people think an average of around 20,00 to 50,000 thoughts a day, but get these statistics: they conclude that 90% of your thoughts are repetitive and—here's the kicker—for most people, over 80% of those thoughts are negative.

Researching information like that, I soon came to understand how important it was that my mindset was established correctly to enable me to obtain my freedom and not remain in a position of being a hostage.

I had fallen into a pattern of entertaining thoughts of fear, loss, and constant danger. In studying how the mind works, I concluded that my thoughts were driven by the mindset that had been established within me. However, the astounding thing was that I was responsible for the mindset being established. Through repetitiously allowing thoughts of fear, loss, and destruction, over time, I created a mindset that determined the attributes of my future thoughts.

Each of us generates thoughts based on the information that we receive from our surroundings; that is, from what we are exposed to. However, the tendency of the type of future thought that you think you will have is influenced and even determined by your mindset.

Since behavioral science has concluded that the way a person thinks will ultimately determine how a person behaves, I have drawn my own conclusions: if someone wants to change the way they behave, they need to change the way they think, so establishing a correct mindset is fundamental.

For myself, because of my belief in God, I began to meditate on the Word of God to reconstruct my mindset. I wanted to be able to think the way God wanted me to think.

> Romans 12:2 (AMP): Do not be conformed to this world (this age), [fashioned after and adapted to its external, superficial customs], but be transformed (changed) by the [entire] renewal of your mind [by its new ideals and its new attitude], so that you may prove [for yourselves] what is the good and acceptable and perfect will of God, even the thing which is good and acceptable and perfect [in His sight for you].

For me, this was it. I wanted change in my life. I didn't want to be held hostage to panic attacks. I wanted to be transformed, and that transformation would occur by the renewal of my mind to the Word of God.

I looked to the Word of God in developing a new mindset, which would be governed by my faith in God.

If you believe in God, this is the route you want to go. If you do not believe in God, you will have to find what works best for you to develop a new mindset.

The encouragement that I would like to instill within you is that I obtained my success through my relationship with God my Father and Jesus my Savior. I want to encourage you to allow God to help you obtain your freedom from panic attacks, anxiety disorder, and any other bondages that you are facing.

Along with Romans 12:2, another verse that helped me to discover the truth is

> Colossians 3:1 – 2 (AMP): The word says – If then you have been raised with Christ [to a new life, thus sharing His resurrection from the dead], aim at and seek the [rich, eternal treasures] that are above, where Christ is, seated at the right hand of God.
>
> And set your minds and keep them set on what is above (the higher things), not on the things that are on the earth.

What caught my attention in this verse was the instruction that I should set my mind on the promises of God, not on all the junk in this world. Okay, that was my start—I was going to establish a new mindset.

UNDERSTANDING THE WAY WE THINK

I want to teach you something that is very vital concerning the relationship of panic attacks with the mindset that becomes established.

Panic disorder, and to some degree, anxiety disorder is just so amazingly tormenting and painful. Because of that, a vicious cycle is established.

For anyone who has ever experienced a panic attack, the biggest thing that you know is that you do not want to have another. Because of that, the normal tendency is to become very watchful and overanalytical in the attempt to ward off another terrifying event.

What I'm saying is that the nature of a panic attack is such that it creates a behavior that will cause a harmful mindset to be established that encourages the onset of future panic attacks.

This revelation was what put me on my path to freedom.

Now, follow me closely. Before I ever experienced a panic attack, I opened the door to become a victim due to the mindset that was established within me over time, years before the first panic attack.

I had a tendency to overanalyze and overthink situations. In the business world, this was a tremendous asset because of the way that I would process things—my thoughts—would enable me to manage restaurants and develop employees very effectively.

One of my strengths was in being extremely perceptive. When I found an employee doing something that they should not be doing, they would often tell me that I had a way of always showing up at the wrong time. However, that wasn't the case—other managers were also in the vicinity. It was just that I was extremely perceptive; I seem to be able to pick up on things that other people are oblivious to.

Although it sounds great and effective, I did not realize that the mindset that I had allowed to develop was one that caused me to be <u>overly watchful</u>.

I would perceive much more than normal, and then would always analyze and overthink. As you read this, I'm sure a lot of you can identify with the tendencies that I had.

When I got hit with my first panic attack, my tendencies went wild. I couldn't wrap my mind around what was happening, but whatever happened, I desperately did not want it to happen again. Thus, the onset of a vicious cycle!

This took me from a vulnerable mindset to a harmful, enabling mindset. I felt so deceived. I'd assumed that the way I was thinking— being overly watchful—was going to help me stop having panic attacks, whereas, in reality, all I did was create a mindset with pom-poms that became a constantly effective cheerleader for future attacks.

I was one of those pain-in-the-butt people who would rarely forget things, like running out of gas or losing the keys or the phone. I've even gone my entire life never getting a speeding ticket. I would like to say that I was just being very responsible, but I found out that my justification for being overly responsible was simply to mask the fact that I worried too much.

The definition of worry is to give way to anxiety or unease by allowing one's mind to dwell on difficulties or potential troubles. Wow, that was me. I would try to mask it by calling myself responsible, but I just plain worried too much.

Normally, these traits are not a huge problem unless they take you to the point where you are susceptible to a panic or anxiety attack. However, for me, the even bigger problem was that these tendencies encouraged the future events of panic attacks instead of helping me war against them.

Panic attacks are very illogical. Because of that, they can be very tormenting. When you overanalyze and overthink, you are always looking for conclusions. Sometimes there is no need for a conclusion, and sometimes there's no conclusion that can be found. My problem is that I would not know when to let things go. Sound familiar to anyone? If you don't let things go, you will train your mind to employ the harmful use of speculation. As we know, speculation is formulating, or attempting to formulate, a conclusion without firm evidence.

Panic disorder is illogical. Panic disorder is not something that you can just wrap your mind around and obtain logical conclusions. Because of my nature, because of my established mindset, something vague and illogical was unacceptable. I was a person who had to have all the answers and who couldn't just let things go. Because of that, I became my own worst enemy. The way I was "wired" encouraged the onset of panic attacks and actually prolonged the duration of the attack.

When this happens to people like me, we become obsessed with overthinking something that is not going to offer a quick conclusion. Unfortunately, this is where a stronghold begins to emerge. A stronghold is a harmful, unwanted pattern of thinking that is the result of overthinking thoughts that now follow the same path. When your mindset encourages continuous thoughts that follow the exact same path, a rut begins to form. Remember the example that I gave you about being in the mountains and following logging trails. This is exactly what happens—you overthink, overanalyze, obsess about your health and how you feel and everything else that can be attributed to a panic attack. This develops one deep rut after another.

The point I am making is that what I was allowing caused the bad to go to worse. My freedom was going to be found in stopping the destructive behavior that I had plunged in to.

Okay, rest your mind for a second, and let me make this a little easier for you with a simple example.

I concluded that my friends would behave differently because they did not think the way I thought. We had a different mindset.

My oblivious friends would feel physically lousy on a certain day. Their response would be, "Wow, I feel lousy. I'm going to make sure I get a good night's sleep tonight so I will feel great tomorrow." Amazingly, most of the time, they would end up feeling great the next day. Just between you and me, sometimes I want to hurt those people. Just kidding. Anyway, my friends and other people I knew were just so quick to be able to let things go.

Not me, I would overanalyze, speculate, and fail to just let things go, especially if it was something to do with my health. If I felt physically lousy there had to be an underlying reason. *I had to have answers, and I had to reach conclusions.* Somewhere, somehow in my life, over time, a unique mindset was allowed to be established, or it would be more accurate to say that I allowed this unique mindset to be established.

With the onset of a panic attack, my cute, little unique mindset shifted to a very harmful mindset. I was standing on a mound of gun powder while playing with matches. *My mindset caused me to over analyze, overthink, demand answers,* and therefore, I fueled the potential for panic attacks through relentless speculation.

When the feelings of a panic attack would hit, remember, I would speculate that I was going to die. I would usually speculate that either I was having a heart attack or that the state that I was in would cause me to have a heart attack.

My friends didn't think this way, so why did I?

THOUGHT BOUNDARIES

In studying what was happening, I began to formulate a line of attack.

Initially, I realized that the pattern of my thoughts established a mindset that channeled future thoughts in an unacceptable direction causing an unacceptable behavior.

To develop a new mindset, I had to censor or restrict entertaining any thoughts that did not line up with how I wanted my future thoughts to be processed. In other words, as stated previously, when I entertained and gave my attention to developing a mindset, the mindset would then influence the formation of my future thoughts.

In the process of creating a new mindset, I found the need to establish mental barriers. I had to figure out how to keep Charlie the goat from breaking out of the pen.

Looking back now, I can see so clearly what was happening to me and where I was making my mistakes. If I would have known then what I know now, I would not have gone through years of torment. This is why it is so important to me that you learn from my vulnerabilities and from my mistakes. If you are being held hostage by panic disorder, I am determined to see you obtain your freedom.

I'm going to lay out very specific tactics that I learned on my journey to freedom. I don't want to get hung up on the exact timeline and the exact order of the tactics that I developed. I just want you to know what I did to obtain freedom so that you can adopt whatever is helpful to you into your life.

What I learned was through trial and error over many years. I also learned through my own experiences and from counseling many people. Initially, I went from fighting to survive to gaining some control to experiencing a few victories and then all the way up to finally obtaining my freedom.

I'm going to attempt to tell you all the things that I have employed to become free, and then I'm going to give you a concise game plan for you to obtain your freedom.

> As we move forward, be very determined
> not to live by your feelings.
> Instead, determine how you want to feel and then become
> very determined to think in line with how you want to feel.
>
> Don't allow your feelings to determine how you think.
> Choose how you WANT TO FEEL.
> Let that determine the WAY YOU MUST THINK.

FIRST AID FOR PANIC ATTACKS

My line of attack

I'm going to give you the details of the path that I took to get free. A lot of what I'm teaching you is what I learned from trial and error. Initially, I did not understand thought patterns, mindsets, strongholds, or any of that junk. I had to learn as I went along. As I tell you the tactics and methods I adopted to overcome panic disorder, you will quickly see how, initially, I was creating a new mindset and setting up thought barriers without even realizing it. Again, I know it was God's help and God's leading that enabled me to defeat this beast.

Okay, enough yakking; let's get moving. The faster you understand the tactics that I used, the faster we will be able to formulate your line of attack. Remember, the timing of each event may not be perfect, but the process that I used is very accurate. On with the show!

LOOKING BACK AT WHERE I STARTED FROM

In the beginning, I was strictly in survival mode. I woke up each morning facing the question of how in the world I was going to make it through the day. The quality of life that I once enjoyed was gone. I was devoid of all stability and any form of peace.

It was very hard for me to eat anything—my stomach was feeling the effects of constant anxiety—and attempting to sleep was a joke. Things got so bad that a lot of nights, I had to sleep outside. For a long time, I would keep waking up at between three and four in the morning and I was tormented for hours about being alone and by runaway thoughts.

For several weeks, I would not even go to bed. I would sit in a lazy boy chair, fully dressed, so that I would be ready to be picked up by the ambulance at a moment's notice. I felt so horrible that I became convinced that I would probably end up in the hospital before the end of the night.

I was quickly beginning to lose all hope. One day, I was walking along the shoulder of the road, watching cars come towards me and fly by. I found myself entertaining the thought that if only a car would veer off the road and hit me, then all this torment would finally go away.

Something had to be done. I'd always believed in God, but now it was time to turn to God to receive my deliverance.

I increased my time in the Word of God and in prayer and came to the conclusion that God would either show me the way out of this or else I was ready to check out and go to Heaven. Either option was fine with me.

In *Hebrews 2:15*, the Word of God says that Jesus delivered and completely set free all those who, through the haunting fear of death, were held in bondage.

I didn't feel like it was time for me to pass on and go to Heaven, so I became committed to obtaining my freedom with the help of God blessing me with wisdom and giving me the determination to break the back of this affliction.

It's one thing to say you're going to trust God and quite another thing to truly walk it out. Gaining trust was a work in progress.

For me, the onset of my panic attacks was so rough because, in the 1990s, there was not any good information available that I could turn to in order to gain some understanding as to what was happening. And on my own, it was hard to just calm down, relax, and approach things logically.

My mind was so consumed with thoughts of fear and death that I could not begin to entertain thoughts that would enable me to see my way out of this. Looking back, this is where I can now see the consequences of a harmful mindset.

Anyway, my initial line of attack:

- I got a physical exam.
- I began to take some medication.
- I became very protective of anything that I heard or anything that I saw. I stopped watching any TV shows concerning drama, especially dramas that dealt with people in medical crises. This is how I began to learn about harmful thought patterns. In any medical crisis, real or fictional, that other people were going through, I found that I would conclude that what was wrong with them was most likely wrong with me also. Any information that I was exposed to had the ability to take me to a devastating conclusion.

  Because I had allowed a harmful mindset to be established within me, that mindset promoted a harmful thought pattern that had the ability to take any tidbit of questionable information and apply it to my life in a negative way by causing me to adopt the thoughts of tragic outcomes based purely on speculation.

  As I began to understand this, I realized that any entertainment that I was exposed to had to be light and comical in nature. Therefore:

- I meditated on the promises of God.

- I made sure that I did not eat or drink anything that had caffeine. The last thing I needed was an extra boost to the excitable state I was already in.
- I enlisted some help from friends. I found that if I engaged people in intentional conversations meant to disrupt my runaway thoughts, the panic attack would not last as long. I also came to understand that if I could cause myself to begin laughing at anything, the flow of adrenaline in my body seemed to quickly subside. I found that I had to get a few people and educate them on how to help me. I needed people who were smart, quick, funny, and very perceptive. This is crucially important. I had to find people who were focused on how important it was that we end the initial panic attack ASAP to stop the flow of adrenaline.
- Next, I determined that if I controlled some of my runaway thoughts, I would begin to shorten the duration of panic attacks, even without the help of other people.

> I had not yet learned how to stop them, but through the help of others, I learned how to shorten the duration and the severity of the attack

Line of Attack – Simplified

1. I got a physical.
2. I began to take meds.
3. I limited any entertainment to good clean comedy.
4. I meditated on the promises of God.
5. I eliminated caffeine from my diet.
6. I found go-to people to help me get through my panic attacks.

BREAKTHROUGH—by controlling some of my runaway thoughts, I began to shorten the duration of panic attacks, even without the help of other people.

OVERCOMING MY BIGGEST OBSTACLE

From the beginning, what I was most obsessed about was my heart. I was convinced that I was going to have a heart attack, either because something was wrong or because of the stress that I was continually putting on my heart from the anxiety and the constant surges of adrenaline that would shoot through my body. I mean, how much could my ticker endure?

I need to interject something here. An intense fear would emerge in me based on what the event of a panic attack would put my body through. As the fear would escalate, I would reach the point where I felt that, if I did not hold on very tight, the mental torment would eventually cause everything to just break apart and fly into little pieces. The physical pain was horrible, but the mental anguish would become unbearable. This is what drove me to my strategic move.

Even though my doctor, Dr. Stratton, concluded that I was physically healthy, I was able to talk him into allowing me to get a cardiac stress test. Just between you and me, the stress test was more for my mind than for my heart. Even though I had a complete physical, I needed further reassurance. We finally got the okay from the insurance company and I was scheduled for what is called a stress/echo.

Basically, you walk on the treadmill until you max out what you feel you can handle. Then they use echo equipment to view the function of your heart and the flow of your blood at maximum production.

FACE TO FACE WITH THE DRILL SERGEANT

Well, I showed up at the cardiac center ready for my little test. While prepping me, the nurse asked why I felt I needed a stress echo. I explained to her that I wanted the peace of mind that everything was working properly. Half-kidding, I told her that I really wanted her to put me through the mill because, when this was over, I wanted to know that everything was good. She gave a little chuckle, and I knew right then that I'd probably made a stupid request. This woman reminded me more of a drill sergeant than someone who specialized in TLC. Not just that, but she also had a certain twinkle in her eye that convinced me that she was going to thoroughly enjoy the pain she was about to put me through.

Typical me, I was being totally held hostage by panic disorder, but I was still able to maintain my competitive spirit. I was on the treadmill for something like 20 to 25 minutes at max pace. I never knew my heart could beat so fast, so loud, and so hard. My breathing was so heavy that I swear the curtains on the windows across the room were flexing to the rhythm of my inhales and exhales.

Just when I reached the point where I was convinced that I was going to collapse, my drill sergeant, sorry, my nurse, screamed out, "Three more minutes, that should do you!"

Three more minutes, are you nuts? I thought. I was sure that I had already begun to hear the angels singing.

Finally, the three minutes were up, and she tossed me from the treadmill onto the examining table as if I were a side of beef in a butcher shop; she was just enjoying this a little too much. By this time, her little cronies were starting the echo and checking everything out. It must be done immediately so they can test you while you are still at your max.

I never knew my heart could beat so fast. The only thing that went through my mind was how far away they stored the shock paddles just in case my heart lost interest in this absurd little experiment.

Finally, we were done. The nurse told me that I had done a really good job. I didn't know if she was referring to the fact that I was in very good shape or to the amount of entertainment that I'd provided for her.

When I left the medical center, I felt different. I knew I would not get the results for a couple of days, but it didn't really matter. I just went through physical stress like I had never experienced before. I knew that by making it through the stress test, I was in no danger from the exertion of a panic attack.

Starting the next day, I began to run and do power walks consistently, making sure that my heart was put through a healthy routine.

I realized that something was different. Some ammunition was taken away from my thought patterns; a mind barrier was put in place. Charlie the goat was made to stay in the pen. I was tempted to tell you that I shot Charlie, but then I figured you might not know that I was kidding and someone would have the animal rights activists pounding at my door by the end of the day.

Again, I just need to interject something here. You must understand; at the time, I did not fully comprehend what I was doing. I did not understand mindsets, thought barriers, and harmful speculation. However, I was starting to develop a new mindset and began to put up mental barriers to corral my continual runaway thoughts.

Something definitely changed after I had my stress echo. The fear of having a heart attack left me. In other words, the fear that fueled the speculation was removed.

With this discovery, I knew that I was onto something here. For the first time, I experienced something positive—a slight breakthrough. This is where I really began to gain an understanding of creating boundaries for my thoughts. Though it was only the beginning, I knew I was headed in the right direction. I realized that I had to have a strong defense so that the goats could not easily escape and do damage. When I look back at how vulnerable I was, not only did I not have a strong fence, but I didn't even have a gate. There was a hole where the gate was supposed to be. My thoughts— "the goats"—had the ability to come and go as they pleased, with no limitations.

Initially, I knew little to nothing about panic attacks. Today, with everything I have learned over the years, I can say that I have learned that panic attacks are caused by:

- The consequences of the unnecessary release of adrenaline into the bloodstream.

- A mindset that encourages overthinking and overanalyzing.
- An overactive negative imagination.
- The adapting of excessive, harmful speculation as a normal way of life.
- Thoughts that have been allowed and trained to operate outside a healthy mental barrier or mindset.

Having told you this information, I will continue to reveal the tactics that I used to overcome my panic attacks. What I did initially had some effect, but again, I continued to learn by trial and error.

It didn't take me long to learn how important it was to attempt to stop a panic attack as fast as possible. The longer I stayed in a panic attack, the more devastating the results were.

The first thing I did was to focus on minimizing the effect of the release of adrenaline into my body. I did not yet have the confidence to stop the release of adrenaline, so the next best thing was to minimize the damage. You minimize the effect by attempting to not overreact to what is happening so that you minimize the fear that you perceive. This is because it's the presence of fear in the mind that prompts the body to release more adrenaline.

I want to make sure that you understand how crucial this is.

What you experience with a panic attack is the unnecessary release of adrenalin. This happens in two ways.

1. Something in your subconscious perceives danger, and therefore, adrenaline is released into your bloodstream even though your conscious mind does not perceive any danger.
2. The tendency to overthink and overanalyze situations and circumstances drives you to a place of being very anxious and stressed out. In this constant state, which is devoid of peace, you become overly watchful and you become very edgy. In this state, you develop nerve sensitization, which causes anything that you feel to be greatly magnified. Constant stress and mental pressure

have the ability to take on the characteristics of danger because of your inability to attempt to control things that are not controllable. Instead of learning to control your reaction to circumstances and situations, you are instead deceived into trying to control any situation and circumstance that you are subject to. What you're trying to do is impossible. Because it is not possible, you experience a sense of failure and a perceived loss of control. Because of that, your mind perceives danger even though, in all actuality, it is only a "self-induced" danger. In this constant state of stress, small levels of adrenaline are released into your bloodstream and continue to build until the adrenaline causes your body to react in a confusing manner, which then has the ability to push you "over the edge" because you have already maxed out what you "feel" you can handle. You attempt to control the situation but cannot because you do not have the ability to "let things go." As a result, you are pushed to the breaking point.

I believe that, for me, both situations that I just mentioned pertained to why I was experiencing the onset of panic attacks.

Let's start with the issue of the subconscious mind perceiving something dangerous that the conscious mind is not aware of. I spent a lot of time in the previous chapters telling you about this, and I'm going to show you the steps that I used to deal with it.

Let me set the stage before I give you my line of attack. One of the most frequent causes for the onset of a panic attack is one's subconscious perception of potential danger. Remember: it's a perception, not an actual danger.

There were certain places and situations that would initiate a panic attack for me. Why? Because it was only a perceived danger by my subconscious and not an understood danger by my conscious mind.

A crucial thing to understand is that your body is trained to release adrenaline into the bloodstream when it receives information from the brain that there is a present danger. Like I said before, the body doesn't sit down and reason with the brain as to the accuracy of the evaluation of the presence of danger; rather, the body only reacts.

If you have struggled with panic attacks long enough, by now you have comprised a list of places or situations that you have found to be unacceptable. For some reason, these places or situations make you feel extremely uncomfortable and can cause you to go into a panic.

This is the hardest thing for somebody to understand who's never had a panic attack. Why? because it's totally illogical. It may be totally illogical, but for some reason, it occurs. Therefore, you must logically attack the illogical.

Over the years, I have had so many couples approach me where one of the spouses would experience panic attacks and the other spouse could just not understand what was going on. They didn't mean to be insensitive; they just couldn't wrap their minds around this illogical reaction to an unknown terror. The information in this book will help to educate people around you about what is going on in your life.

Okay, for whatever reason, these are some of the situations that made me uncomfortable and, therefore, unacceptable.

- Large stores, particularly the one in which I would always get my groceries.
- Driving on crowded highways.
- Driving on roads where I had to drive down steep inclines.
- Being a passenger on a crowded bus or crowded cars.
- Any large building where I was far from the exit.
- The preparation for going on the trip.
- Business meetings where I didn't have the freedom to just up and leave.
- Being isolated from people that I knew well.
- Being in a remote area, far away from potential medical help.

Don't waste your time trying to figure out why something causes your subconscious to view that something as being dangerous. What we are going to spend our time on is how to re-educate the subconscious.

The lesson that I learned from obtaining a stress echo was that I was able to eliminate some obsessive negative patterns.

Without knowing it, I was developing a new mindset by forcing myself to focus on what I wanted to think about instead of what I was trained to think about.

Without knowing it, I was developing mental barriers for my thought patterns. After the stress echo, I ruled out the speculation that I was going to have a heart attack. That thought, "that goat," was never going to be allowed to leave the pen again. From that point on, I was determined never to meditate on the possibility that I was going to have a heart attack. Sounds trite and trivial, but it was a huge step for me.

I was on the right track and could smell success, so I continued on my way.

I had some other "goats" that spent a lot of time outside of the pen, and that was unacceptable. One thing that I cannot understand is why I began to have a fear of going to the local grocery store. There was no reason for it, and that's exactly why I decided to tackle it. Remember, don't waste your time looking for reasons; invest your time finding solutions.

Why did my subconscious view the grocery store as uncomfortable, as a place of danger? Well, it didn't matter why, but I was determined to put an end to it.

At this point, I was out of the survival mode, and I was setting up some strong defenses. I became stronger by:

- Meditating on the Word of God.
- Speaking statements of truth over my life.
- Learning the value of laughter to stop the flow of adrenaline.

- Learning how to take thoughts captive.
- Learning the importance of go-to people.

I quickly learned that, not only did I have to be equipped with defenses, but; I also had to start going on the offense. I made up my mind to tackle the grocery store and dispel whatever danger my subconscious was perceiving.

My preparation for hitting the grocery store was developing a stronger positive mindset, gaining the confidence found from taking thoughts captive, and realizing the importance of speaking out loud to stop runaway thoughts.

I entered the grocery store and basically did the opposite of what I did when I was taken off guard and held hostage. My tactics:

- I did not allow myself to entertain any negative thoughts.
- I engaged people in conversation to disrupt any negative thought patterns.
- I spoke words of faith out loud.
- If I felt anything negative, I spoke the opposite of what I felt.
- I forced myself to chuckle and laugh. I began to laugh at myself about how silly the way I felt before was.

For my first *"Let's go on the offensive"* attack, I didn't spend a ton of time in the store; rather, I simply got my shopping done and left. To this day, it's a mystery that I couldn't have cared less about what it was that I purchased—I was not there to stock my shelves and look for bargains; I was there to turn the tables on panic attacks I'd suffered for so long.

For years, my panic attacks had been attacking me, and for the first time, I was in the process of attacking the panic attacks back. Amazingly, I was successful. I entered a situation that before was perceived by my subconscious to be a threat, but I endured the experience without any feelings of fear or being uncomfortable.

This is huge and you have to get this. What I accomplished was to prove to my subconscious that there was no danger.

Whenever my subconscious perceived danger and I supported the perception, adrenaline was released, and I had a panic attack. When I refused to support a harmful perception of my subconscious, there was no perception of danger, there was no fear, and there was no release of adrenaline.

The next day, I went to the store, even though I did not need anything, and went through the same procedure. I spent much more time in the store than was needed, and I spent most of the time as far away from the exit doors as possible. When I went to check out, I picked the line that was the longest.

What I did was to do the exact opposite of the tendencies I'd had before. Why? so I could prove that I was in no danger so the need for speculation was never initiated.

This is amazing, I thought. I realized that I was starting to go on the offense.

For anyone who has never experienced a panic attack, the hype of this whole procedure probably seems absurd. That's okay. If I'd never had a panic attack, I'm sure that I would be chuckling right along with you.

I need you to understand that before I ever had a panic attack episode, I was viewed as being extremely logical and down to earth. I believe that is why what I went through was so hard for other people to understand. I know it was completely baffling to me. I don't deal with the illogical very well. Let me tell you about an episode that I experienced just to help you understand how powerful the subconscious can be.

I have divided my battle with panic attacks into sections. We had survival mode, defensive/maintenance mode, going on the offensive/attack mode, and finally, obtaining freedom while keeping a very watchful eye.

The story that I'm telling you took place after having passed through the defensive/maintenance mode and while I was well into the offensive/ attack mode. This is probably around five to seven years after the initial onset of my panic attacks. Anyway, one day, I was driving down the road when I suddenly became very uncomfortable and a blast of fear and confusion attempted to overtake me. I could feel the release of adrenaline start to impact my body.

Because of all the steps that I had adopted getting to this point of being able to control an oncoming panic attack, I did not allow the panic attack to take place. Refusing to give in to speculation and confusion, I spoke words of faith and words of truth out loud, and within no time at all, the attempted attack was well under control.

I continued driving, and everything returned to a normal, relaxed state. I did not overanalyze. I knew what had happened; I just didn't know in this case why it had happened.

Later that same day, I finally received the understanding. I remembered that, several years ago, I'd had a brutal panic attack at that very spot on the road I was now traveling. It was on the crest of a steep hill. For some reason, when I was initially in bondage to my panic attacks, I felt it very difficult to travel down steep inclines while driving. For some reason, back in the early stages of my panic attacks, when I was in survival mode, this exact point of the road triggered one of the most horrifying attacks that I had ever experienced.

The point I want you to receive from this experience is just how powerful the subconscious can be. When I approached the part of the road that initiated the panic attack years ago, I had absolutely no awareness and no consciousness that driving down that very steep incline would ever, or should ever, be a problem. In my conscious mind, I was totally comfortable and perceived absolutely no apprehension about traveling that road. However, because I had experienced such a severe panic attack some years before at that spot, my subconscious was able to store the memory of the experience, and it was powerful enough to initiate the perception of danger without my conscious awareness having any idea of what was going on.

If I had not intentionally worked to change my mindset and disrupt the harmful patterns that I once had, I could have easily fallen victim to another vicious panic attack. However, the potential panic attack could not gain momentum because I took away its fuel (i.e., speculation). As soon as I realized that my subconscious still perceived a danger, I traveled back to that spot the next day. As I traveled down the steep incline approaching the spot, I could still feel a slight bit of apprehension. So, I turned around and traveled the path again. I repeated the process two more times until I was completely comfortable with traveling over that section of the road. The process that I was applying was that of reeducating my subconscious.

To tell a story like this has the potential to make me feel embarrassed— wrestling with such a pathetically trite accomplishment. However, this is one of the keys to understanding panic attacks.

If I was parachuting out of an airplane, scaling down the face of a steep mountainside, or bungee jumping off a bridge over a gorge, the fear and the apprehension would all be logical. On the other hand, having a fear of driving down a steep hill on a highway is completely illogical. If you start out by beating yourself up for the way you feel, you will just add to the anxiety of the beast of panic disorder.

Panic attacks must be fueled by an illogical fear, or there would be no need for speculation. If I am about to be shoved out of a plane with the hope of parachuting safely to the ground, I'm going to feel fear. I get it; that's logical. There's nothing more to think about. They slap a parachute on you and kick you out of the plane after they have pried your white-knuckled grip from the edges of the door, kicking and screaming all the way down until you safely reach the ground. After you tuck and roll and do a face plant in the dirt, the fear is gone, and you strut around like a proud rooster for having so bravely accomplished such a feat. Put all the kicking and screaming aside and the only thing that is left in your mind is that you "nailed it."

Unfortunately, after I conquered the incline of the road with my vehicle, there were not a lot of cheering fans at the bottom of the incline chanting my name and preparing to hoist me up on their shoulders and parade me around for the photographers.

That's okay because the victory that you achieve by dispelling and conquering a fear that your subconscious is attempting to hold onto, for someone who is inflicted by panic attacks, is just as impressive as something like skydiving.

If you have a spouse who is wrestling with trivial obstacles that initiate fear driven by their subconscious, don't try to understand it—learn how to get them through it. If you're going to beat panic attacks, you better learn how to logically embrace the illogical.

Don't be embarrassed, don't beat yourself up, and learn to face your fear until that fear backs down and leaves you alone.

For a lot of you, the best thing that could've happened to you is to have a completely logical person like me fall prey to and then conquer something that is beyond simple reasoning.

When you are prepared to logically face the illogical and determined to defeat it by making the illogical logical, then you are well on your way to getting a handle on this tormenting beast.

Summary – steps to breakthrough:

- **I identified situations and circumstances that subconsciously I perceived to be dangerous. The reason I knew it was a subconscious fear is that the fear was illogical to my conscious rational thinking.**
- **I began to go on the offensive, to experience these situations and circumstances without the perception of fear, to prove to my subconscious that they were not dangerous.**
- **To accomplish this, I used all the tactics that I previously discussed. I was using the formation of a new mindset, and**

I was starting to establish new thought patterns. I used the process of taking harmful negative thoughts captive by speaking words out loud that opposed those thoughts, while I also refused to feed and strengthen negative thoughts by entertaining them. I meditated on the Word of God to develop my faith in the promises of God to enable me to overcome unwanted fear.

Through my trial-and-error approach to defeating the panic attacks that plagued my life, I finally began to understand which methods were effective and which were not.

For myself, I knew I was dealing with the improper and unnecessary release of adrenaline into my bloodstream, which initially had the ability to really cause confusion and the onset of fear. Along with that, a harmful mindset was developed through continuously harmful patterns of thought.

For some of you, the inappropriate and unneeded release of adrenaline may play a big part in the suffering that you are experiencing. However, for some of you, the daily mental torment of runaway, uncontrollable thoughts producing relentless and debilitating anxiety may be the bigger issue. In either case, the techniques and procedures that I adopted in my deliverance will offer you the same opportunity for success.

So far in this chapter, I have shown you how I went from survival mode to a defensive mode, to where I started to go on the offensive.

As I obtained success in slowing down the inappropriate, unnecessary release of adrenaline and as I learned to reduce the effect that the presence of adrenaline would have on me, I began to focus more and more on reconstructing my thought patterns.

At this point on my path to freedom, I began to learn more about the importance of my mindset and my thought patterns. This was prompted by my need to understand why I was more susceptible to panic attacks and anxiety disorder than others were.

As I stated before, I knew that I was more perceptive than a lot of people. Also, I knew that I had a tendency to overthink and overanalyze things. However, in observing different kinds of people, I realized that there were a lot of people out there who were very perceptive and who also, to a certain degree, engaged in overthinking and overanalyzing things. So, what was up? What was different concerning me that made me susceptible to panic attacks when these other people were not?

This sent me on my path to drawing the conclusion that the way I would think would hinder the way I ultimately wanted to behave. This was going to be absolutely essential. Also, analyzing is great if you need to obtain specific information; however, endless overanalyzing would have to result in relying on speculation, which, in my case, I knew was not acceptable.

So, I began to adopt some techniques to help me acquire the behavioral changes that I was looking for. I knew that the way that I would think would ultimately determine the way I would behave. Therefore, I knew I had to continue to establish new thought patterns and establish a mindset that would support those thought patterns.

"NUTRITION" FOR HEALTHY THOUGHT PATTERNS

MAINTENANCE

If we correlated panic attacks with the health of your body, we could say that the previous chapter would be our emergency first aid kit and the current chapter would be somewhat that of nutrition for the body.

In the last section, I explained how I got out of a survival mode. The next step is how to focus on tactics that, when employed effectively, create an atmosphere that frees you from panic attacks.

As stated before, I was very aware of my heightened perceptiveness, as well as my tendency to overthink and overanalyze. That just did not seem to be enough to trigger panic attacks because many people have these same tendencies. There must have been more to it than that, perhaps a flaw in my thinking pattern that opened the door to panic attacks? The flaw needed to be corrected, but changing any of my core values was not an option.

Being in the hospitality industry, I managed a large staff of over 100 employees. While laying out the groundwork to lessen my vulnerability to panic attacks, I wanted to make sure that any changes made concerning my mindset and thought pattern would not lessen my ability to be effective at work. The staff considered me to be very responsible, a go-to person. They believed I had a gift at counseling others on how to make a positive impact on the lives of my employees.

With that introduction, I am going to continue to reveal the road I traveled to obtain my freedom. At this point in my storyline, we are probably 8—10 years past the initial onset of panic attacks.

I was no longer held hostage to that engulfing, terrifying panic attack that had plagued me the first seven years, but I was still not at a place of freedom that would guarantee me no future panic attacks. At this point, they were not as severe, and their duration was much shorter. However, the potential for a full-blown panic attack was ever-present, like a cloud that seemed to hang over me. Would I ever be vulnerable enough to slide back into the state of despair that I was once held captive to?

I began to understand how effective it was to begin to take back the territory that my panic attacks had been able to rob me of. Starting slowly, I subjected myself to circumstances and situations that, in the past, I'd found to be very uncomfortable, for example, my bold trip to revisit the grocery store to let my mind know who was boss. This method was extremely effective.

In observing other people and having conversations with them, I came to realize that many people seldom had their thoughts go to places where all my thoughts went: impending doom. The conclusion: most people weren't doing anything particularly right; it was just that I was perhaps "allowing" fear and speculation to run rampant in my mind.

And so, it began. I learned how to take thoughts captive by speaking words of faith and truth that opposed negative or harmful thoughts. My coveted freedom would be within reach if only I could understand and control the mind barrier. It is crucial to block pathways to stop runaway thoughts that have the ability to fuel panic attacks and instead replace the negative with peace, joy, and contentment.

During this time, after the onset of panic attacks, my relationship with God continued to increase. However, in my heart, I knew there was more. I needed a closer relationship with God to get me to freedom. I was determined to keep pressing in to the Word of God to gain more revelation.

As is typical for so many people, we tend to trust God the most when we run out of options. Why is that? I was learning more and more about trusting God, but I knew that I had not yet established complete dependency on Him.

In the Bible, the book of Proverbs is the wisdom of God. I knew I needed wisdom, and I knew I needed to learn to continue to increase my trust and faith in Him.

Proverbs 3:5 – 6 was a real eye-opener for me. The verse reads:

> **Proverbs 3:5-6 (NKJV): Trust in the Lord with all your heart and lean not on your own understanding; in all your ways acknowledge Him, and he shall direct your paths.**

Wow, that sounds wonderful. It's one thing to acknowledge the Scripture and it's another thing to live by. Let me paraphrase it the way most of us tend to apply this Scripture:

> *Trust in the Lord with all your heart when you completely run out of options, and lean not to your own understanding after everything else that you tried has failed; acknowledge Him when you have really messed up and you need someone to get you out of your mess, and allow God to direct your paths when you are sure that He will be in complete agreement with the game plan that you have devised.*

So, why is it so hard for us to trust God? I determined in my heart to start applying the Word of God with no strings attached, with no disclaimers.

I will cover this in more depth once the groundwork has been laid. At this point, while studying the Scriptures, I discovered more and more that the Word of God continuously guides us to roll our cares over on Him. Looking back, it was easy to conclude that, not only did I fail to roll my cares over on God, but I also lived a life where I fabricated potential cares to care about. I was a caring machine. Not the noble kind of care, where a person looks out for the welfare of others, but the unintentional selfish cares that surfaced due to the fact that I was driven to entertain more complex and haunting thoughts than was the norm for most others, and in doing so, I was an artist at living by speculation. No one had to tell me to be careful because care was one thing that I knew I was full of.

Of course, I had to ask myself—was it care, or was it worry? Was I living to be responsible, or was I living anxiously because what I chose to be responsible for was more than I was required to carry?

It takes a lot of work to run the world. I should know because, for many years, I attempted to fulfill that job description. Be honest; there must be a lot of you out there attempting to do the same thing.

What I finally began to understand is that I am not responsible for everything that happens around me. I cannot control everything that happens, everything that I am exposed to, but I am responsible for controlling my response to what is going on around me. It's not the circumstance that can defeat you; it's the incorrect response to a circumstance that gets you into trouble.

As I continue with my story, conveying to you the actions I took in defeating my panic attacks, you will begin to understand how I acquired the revelations that I now walk in.

As I stated, at this point in my journey, I knew that I was no longer in survival mode and that I had made good progress in learning how to fight against my panic attacks by applying the wisdom of God. I knew I was still not at the place of healing and freedom that I was convinced was available.

Over the 10 to 12 years after my initial panic attack, my mind really took a beating. The early years were the most harmful and tormenting, and throughout the latter years, I was slowly gaining success against my panic attacks, yet an anxious state remained. Nonetheless, it did not take me to the place of mental strength and mental health that I knew was possible.

So, what exactly went wrong to open the door for my panic attacks? This was a question that I was finally able to ask myself since the bulk of my mental energy was no longer consumed by fighting for survival. I began to scrutinize my past in order to hopefully obtain additional insight so that I could proceed from a state of mere survival to freedom.

TIMELINE OF EVENTS

LIFE BEFORE 1992

To help you out, here's a timeline that will make it a little easier for you to follow.

TIMELINE OF EVENTS

- 1981 – 1992: After graduating from Penn State University, I worked in the restaurant business for 11 years. In all that time, I never missed a day of work. I never had a sick day.
- **May 1992: I experienced my first panic attack.**
- May 1992 – 1999: I was able to do my job, but I was held hostage by fear during this time period. I continued to get beaten up by panic attacks.
- 1999 – 2004: I began to obtain certain levels of success in dealing with panic attacks, but I knew there was so much more for me to learn.
- 2004 – 2008: I received more revelations about the way I processed thoughts, enabling me to make the necessary changes.
- 2008 – present: freedom, and effectiveness.
- 2015 – 2019: devoted time to writing this book to serve as a pathway for others to obtain their freedom.

CATCHING UP ON THE BACK STORY

As I look back over my life, my high school years were quite typical. I received average grades. I knew I had the potential to get better grades, but the presence of low-to-average motivation resulted in nearly average grades.

I never got into any big trouble—no drugs, drinking, or smoking. I was mostly seen but not heard. I got along well with people, and I did whatever it took to blend in. I had no desire whatsoever to stand out from the crowd.

Since I lived in Pennsylvania, I opted to go to Penn State University. Wow, quite a shell shock from high school. Classrooms of up to 500 people. It certainly wasn't like the old TV show "*Cheers,*" where, according to the theme song, "Everybody knows your name." The professors didn't care who you were or even if you showed up or not. You were a number, and how you did on the tests fully determined your standing. There was certainly no sense in wasting any money on buying apples to get in good with the professors. Besides, apples would not have cut it. For those stuffed-shirt teachers, it would have at least taken an investment into a Starbucks latte if you were even going to get their attention. (If Starbucks had existed back then.)

My first year at Penn State was a joke. I was so naïve that I spent the first two weeks waiting for the professor to pass out the textbooks. No one bothered to tell me that you had to buy them yourself. What did I know; I was just a dumb hick from rural Lancaster County.

Sometime towards the end of my first year at Penn State, I finally came to the revelation that if I did not do something soon, I was going to just get trampled by the crowd. Not sure exactly why, but I went from being a person with low to average motivation to a person who was obsessed with excelling at everything.

After my first term, I never missed being on the dean's list. My new-found motivation was to keep my grade point average at 4.0.

During high school, I had become involved in track and gymnastics. Not for the reasons of talent or motivation, but mostly because that's what my friends did.

At Penn State, I had a real desire to become involved in sports. I was certainly not good enough to compete against the high-quality athletes at Penn State, so I pursued just being involved in any way that I could.

By this point, I'd developed firmly into an overachiever. I answered an ad that requested people to help set up for gymnastics meets. Basically, I moved equipment and chairs around; well, there was no challenge and definitely no gratification in doing that.

I had a basic knowledge of gymnastics, and I proceeded to get my hands on anything I could in order to learn the skills of the sport. At this point, being a pain- in- the- butt little overachiever, I weaseled my way into being a type of manager for the things that the team needed.

Well, before I knew it, I'd worked my way up to being somewhat indispensable. I did whatever needed to be done, and I did it well. They began to ask me to help be a "spotter" for the gymnasts while they were practicing. Basically, a "spotter" is someone who is responsible for catching the gymnasts when they lose their grip and fall off the equipment. I was six feet tall, and I had lifted weights ever since high school. I was quick, aware, and very perceptive. I was in the right place at the right time. I made some great "saves" by catching the athletes as they unintentionally went flying off the equipment.

I became obsessed with achieving excellence. Low to average was no longer going to cut it for me; I wanted to be the go-to person and I got my wish. During my senior year, the United States men's gymnastics team trained at Penn State in preparation for the Olympic Games. I did so well that even athletes on the Olympic gymnastics team asked for my help to keep them safe and prevent them from getting hurt.

I had an amazing time, and I became addicted to being the go-to person. I did so well that the athletics department offered me a full scholarship to stay in college and get my doctorate degree so that I would be able to continue to help with the team.

However amazing that offer was, I felt it was time for me to get out and get to work. I was tired of being broke.

Out of college, having a business degree, and specializing in the hospitality industry, I took a job helping a gentleman get a newly purchased restaurant open. Within the few first months, two of the managers that he hired had bailed out on him and he asked me to run the restaurant for him.

Over the next several years, he purchased four more restaurants. Eventually, I was responsible for overseeing all of them.

Then the first panic attack happened. So, once the dust finally settled from the stage of encountering this debilitating panic attack, I began to question myself concerning my life, how the door was opened, and what made me susceptible.

RECAP:

I was conditioned to handle responsibility, pressure, and stress. I had a very enjoyable and successful time during my college years. No regrets, and I remained very content.

During my years at Penn State, I achieved much more than I initially anticipated. I traveled with the college gymnastics team and was responsible for logistics and financial transactions.

After college, I worked my way up to overseeing five restaurants, which were organized and successful. At this point, I was responsible for well over 200 employees.

So, what was the issue? How did I go from being so capable of handling such demanding tasks and responsibility before being brought down to a place of such ineffectiveness to where I was defeated by simple things like buying groceries and traveling down steep inclines in my vehicle?

I continued to search for answers. Not in a harmful, obsessive way; I just wanted, needed, logical answers for what had happened so that I would be less susceptible to the undesirable happening in the future. In the search for answers, through trial and error, I was blessed to discover tactics that were effective.

SELF-ANALYSIS AND SPIRITUAL GROWTH

As I continue my story, I would estimate that we are probably just at the turn of the century, probably around 2001.

At this point, I found myself searching for deeper answers to why this happened to me, searching for any necessary changes in how I handled everyday situations.

During this time, I began to spend more and more time ministering to other people who were being beaten up by panic attacks. My main objective was that I just did not want to see people in such torment. Along with that, the need to be a go-to person would tend to surface, in a good way. Also, I realized that, in helping people, I was gaining more and more insight into finding ways to serve as a preventative for initial and future attacks. During this time, my faith in God and my dependency on Him continued to grow. The Word of God gave me insight into how to correctly and effectively live. There were a few very crucial revelations from the Word of God that I relied on to obtain understanding about panic attacks. We will do a comprehensive study of this beginning in chapter 18. But I've just a few things I want to mention here to help you understand the importance of the next steps that we will be taking.

First, it is important to understand that we are spirit beings. The Bible says that we are made in the image and likeness of God.

Second, we have a realm called the soul. The soul is comprised of the mind, the will, and the emotions.

Third, the spirit and the realm of the soul are housed in a body.

When God created the Earth, it was devoid of evil; therefore, there was no knowledge of evil. When the enemy successfully deceived Adam and Eve, a knowledge of evil was now released into the Earth and a curse came upon the Earth.

The Word of God says:

> John 10:10 (NKJV): The thief, the enemy comes to kill, steal, and destroy. Jesus came so that we could have life and have it in abundance.

Well, I can tell you that, for many years, I was not enjoying the abundant life that Jesus came to provide for me.

The Word of God tells us:

> Ephesians 6:12 (NKJV): We wrestle not with flesh and blood, but against principalities, against powers, against the rulers of the darkness of this age, against spiritual hosts of wickedness in the heavenly places.

CONCLUSIONS:

I know that God is my Father, Jesus is my Savior, and I am filled with the Holy Spirit. The Holy Spirit leads me to truth.

We have an enemy; it is the demonic realm. The battleground is in the realm of our soul. The demonic realm has the ability to attack our thoughts and our emotions in an effort to drive evil, demonic behavior. In other words, the devil does not have the ability to destroy us; rather, the enemy must use deceptive tactics to attack our mind to cause us to self-destruct.

Okay, back to the storyline. As I said, we are somewhere around 2000 to 2002, when I decided to invest my time and energy into understanding why I was so susceptible to panic attacks. Also, I wanted more insight so I could be more effective at helping other people who were struggling. By this time, I knew that there was a strong probability that, one day, I would be writing a book about panic attacks. Anyway, for all the reasons above, I persisted in order to solve the mystery.

By this time, I had a pretty firm understanding of what panic attacks were and how they functioned to cause such pain and suffering, but still, the question just would not go away. Why me? I mean, come on, I was good at what I did.

So, what was it that I had done so repetitively over the years? I managed, I maintained, and I was responsible for people—mostly for their safety.

As I continued to question myself, I began to see a pattern that was emerging. I was a maintainer. I was not an innovator, not an inventor—no, I was a maintainer.

Since I was always called to maintain things that caused me to be "wired" a certain way or because I was "wired" a certain way, did that mean I always gravitated towards maintaining?

I realized that, since childhood, I had to be responsible for the health and the safety of people around me. In high school, I remember being the one who would always encourage people to put safety first as they developed their gymnastic skills. I remembered that I would take on the responsibility to closely watch someone when they were doing their gymnastics routine if I knew they were going to do something difficult.

In college, I became directly responsible for the safety of people who had spent most of their lives working towards their upcoming Olympic opportunity. People who train for the Olympics often have over 12 years invested in this one opportunity for success.

As I was reflecting on this, I began to remember just how much responsibility I felt for keeping people safe.

Then I transitioned to the hospitality industry. For most people, running a single restaurant is a nightmare. I was overseeing five restaurants. The responsibility for food safety was never-ending, but that was maintenance. I loved to maintain—I was "wired" to maintain.

A pattern was beginning to emerge. Even as a child, I took the responsibility to maintain. I remember when I and the other ornery young kids would engage in accepting dares and taking risks that were a normal part of growing up, I would be an ever-present reminder of efforts to ensure safety.

THE ICY SLED RUN

I remember when I was about 10 years old, a gang of us would often sled during the winter. We lived in a little development and would always look for steep hills to turn into sledding runs. One of the kids in our gang had a dad who was on the borough crew for our town. We would harass and nag the poor man until he would finally let us put up "road closed except for local traffic" signs. There was one steep hill that we would always use. Before we went home at night after a day of fun, we would carry water out to pour on our snowy road to make a sheet of ice to ensure high speed sledding for the next day. You had to know what you were doing if you chose to take the challenge to sled down our hill.

As was so typical for me, I demanded that we put some straw bales at the bottom of the hill and that we would pile a lot of loose snow in front of the straw bales so that we would always be able to stop before we ended up wrapping our sleds around a tree or catapulting our heads through somebody's fence. I remember some of the most fun we had was when kids from different neighborhoods would venture into our area and had the nerve to ask if they could sled down our hill. We would always say yes, and we would always gather together at the top of the hill to watch for the predictable outcome of screams of terror culminating in one big explosive puff of snow and straw as, inevitably, a new kid would go crashing into the barrier.

So, as I was putting all this information together, sometime around 2001, I suddenly realized that I always focused on maintaining and encouraging safety. That was my mindset, which produced patterns of thinking that most always entertained thoughts of safety and things running correctly.

When we were kids, seeking the thrill of sledding, the more we traveled the same path for sledding on the same hill, the more that path got more packed down and we would travel faster and faster. Amazingly, that sledding track reflected my thought pattern.

You see, through my childhood, high school days, college days, and even with my career choice, all things involved safety. But here's the amazing revelation that brought on and invited speculation. Not only did I make myself responsible for the safety of the obvious, but I also made myself responsible for continuously meditating on scenarios of potential danger so that I would be prepared with a safety plan.

In my efforts to be effective, I drove myself to not only maintain safety in the things I saw, as stated above, but I also drove myself to speculate on every possible scenario of things that could go wrong so that I would already have a safety measure for all possible situations.

My thought pattern was like a well-iced, well-traveled sledding run. Unfortunately, I never took the time to put a barrier on my thought patterns as I so carefully did on our sledding run, where I made sure we had the safety of a barrier of snow and straw bales.

As a "professional" maintainer during my life up to this point, I allowed myself to develop a dependency on speculation. As I stated earlier, there's a fine line between being responsible and engaging in constant unnecessary worry that can turn into harmful anxiety.

Without being aware, I discovered my constant use of speculation was a major cause of the problem. Over the last 10 or 12 years since my first panic attack, I started reducing my use of speculation because I became painfully aware of how harmful it could be. However, with the revelation of what I was learning by reviewing my life to attempt to find answers, it became obvious that my mindset and thought patterns were always strongly embedded with speculation. This is most likely what positioned me to be such a prime candidate for panic attacks.

It was interesting to conclude that I was so good at managing everything— except the vulnerabilities of my own mind.

I had made a lot of changes since my first panic attack that were extremely beneficial. All the same, I had been able to effectively manage and maintain people and business operations throughout the years of dealing with my panic attacks. This was an area of accomplishment, for I did not employ the harmful use of speculation. It took a while for me to understand why.

With managing people, I was effective because of systems that I made sure were in place. The systems left no room for speculation and I now understood that, in order to properly manage my mind, I would have to adopt new methods to obtain the success that I wanted. I had to put similar systems in place to control my susceptibility for overthinking and runaway thoughts.

In this book, I believe that I have provided you with the necessary information on how to reduce the number of panic attacks and their severity. In a later chapter, I will provide you with a very concise "go to" guideline to again remind you exactly what to do at the onset of a panic attack.

However, to further ensure your long-term freedom, we're going to learn some simple techniques to make sure that our mind is developed to work *for* us instead of against us.

As we begin this process, I think it would be beneficial for you to look back on your life, as I did, to see if you can detect possible patterns of harmful thinking that may have been allowed to develop.

There is a close relationship between panic disorder and anxiety disorder. It's amazing how many people in the United States suffer from anxiety; the percentage is very high. It is essential to grasp what in your life might have opened the door to panic attacks and to unhealthy harmful levels of anxiety. So, let's revisit this information.

Anxiety: a feeling of worry, nervousness, or unease, typically about an imminent event or something with an uncertain outcome.

Speculation: the forming of a theory or idea without firm evidence.

What I was exposed to and the responsibilities that I adopted caused me to live by speculation. I would conduct myself in anticipation that something was going to happen, even though there was no firm evidence to support it.

Because of that, without realizing it, I lived in a constant state of anxiety. I was not only concerned about what was happening, but I would also invest care and concern in things that only had a slight potential of happening. Because of this, I gave my mind way too much to be responsible for.

With the first panic attack, I was a prime candidate to be a victim of this disorder. Panic attacks are fed by fear, which is fed by speculation, which, in turn, creates an unbearable amount of anxiety.

Before I ever had a panic attack, there did not seem to be a big problem with my mindset or my thought patterns. However, when a panic attack hit, it was like a sled on that icy path, and there was no barrier to stop the sled, which represented my thoughts. Amazingly, my tendency to overspeculate put one sled after another at the top of the icy path. Each sled represents a thought that went to a very negative, harmful spot and went there extremely fast.

The first thing that I did once I realized what was happening was to begin to strengthen my mind by restricting negative thoughts and thoughts that were prompted by speculation.

I had already begun to develop a healthier mindset and the process of taking thoughts captive. This is what brought my initial success in fighting panic attacks and enabled me to come out of survival mode. At this point in my life, around the year 2001, I came to the conclusion that there was more work to do to develop my mind to obtain the behavior I desired.

In the earlier chapters, I revealed to you how I restricted what I watched and what I listened to. Now I'm going to lay out my attack to further strengthen my mind.

Initially, as I told you, I stopped watching any horror shows or movies and I stopped watching any TV medical dramas. Now I also made the decision not to watch or listen to any news programs. This may sound drastic, and you will have to decide what is right for you, but as for me, I knew that I was driven to always try to fix things, whether it was feasibly possible or not.

Because of that, I had to limit any negative information that I was exposed to on a regular basis. I realized that the more information I entertained would increase the thoughts that I would take on and feel responsible for maintaining.

I replaced most of the information and entertainment that I was exposed to in the past and now limited it to the Word of God and good clean comedy.

Anything that I was exposed to, I was driven to attempt to maintain. Therefore, I had to limit myself to less and less information.

I very intentionally identified and rejected speculation. Remember, my vulnerability was that I would not only deal with what was in front of me, but I would also have to deal with things that could possibly materialize in the future. That's too much! As a drastic action, I began to attempt to slow my thinking down. As things slowed down, I was able to identify what thoughts were purely based on speculation. When I would detect speculation, I would make the following statement: "That's speculation and I will not entertain that thought." The Word of God teaches the benefits of speaking words of faith out loud, and behavioral science is finally catching up and now recognizes the benefits to the brain when words are spoken out loud.

Intentionally, I reduced any thought patterns that would cause me to enter into unnecessary worry or uneasiness. And thus, I began to teach myself how to be responsible while at the same time avoiding worry and stress.

These initial steps eventually directed me to something very vital. I learned to correctly and effectively employ the use of my imagination. While involved in college gymnastics, the value of imagination became a foundation upon which to springboard to success.

Let me explain.

When a gymnast would receive an injury that prevented them from physically being able to practice, they would quickly lose ground and be less competitive. We adopted a technique of going through gymnastics skills and routines in the gymnast's mind, using their imagination. They would sit and, in their mind's eye, visualize their routines in detail. It is amazing the benefit this technique had on increasing the skills of the gymnast, even without physically performing the routines and skills. I had no idea that, years later, I would now be adopting the benefits that I had previously learned about the imagination.

It has been proven and widely accepted that when the imagination is used effectively and with enough repetition, the body loses the ability to discern whether the action took place or was just perceived in the imagination.

This is very important, so try to follow closely. When people employ the use of their imagination, it can either be very beneficial or very harmful.

In my case, without knowing it, in my attempts to be responsible, I would allow my imagination to continuously go to the worst-case scenario so that I could be prepared to deal with situations correctly; that is, if these catastrophes ever happened. It sounds so innocent and harmless. This was the incorrect use of my imagination that would be the driving force to indulging in the use of speculation.

Do you see what was happening to me? I would allow and even prompt my imagination to continuously embrace and meditate on the worst-case scenarios. Wow, it is no wonder that my thoughts would continually go to and live in places that the thoughts other people had would never even stop off for a quick visit.

This was such a huge revelation for me. Every time I entertained a possibility, my imagination was fully prepared to explore the most bizarre, potentially devastating outcomes. Do you see why the onset of my panic attacks found me prepared to be such an excellent victim? On the surface, I was not a negative, doom and gloom type of person, but residing inside my mind was a monster that I allowed to be created. I provided all the fuel that a panic attack would ever need to burn. All that had to happen was the introduction of the first spark and we were off to the races. My mind was like a well-iced sledding path that allowed thoughts to race and encounter extremes.

This was the missing link that I had been searching for. Like I told you before, I always noticed that my friends would not entertain thoughts that I entertained. They were not great maintainers, but most of them had no trouble navigating through life. Sure, maybe they were oblivious, but they also never experienced the torment that I was susceptible to.

And what about all those other people who are victims of panic attacks. They surely don't all become vulnerable through the path of being an obsessive maintainer. No, as I sought for the common denominator, I determined that the imagination was a key proponent, but what a person chose to meditate on would be the deciding factor.

Statistics show us that people entertain anywhere from 20,000 to 60,000 thoughts a day. Remember, we went over the numbers that show that the bulk of many people's thoughts are negative and are repetitive.

In reviewing the people I counseled over the years concerning panic attacks, I could see that many them tended to have some very similar characteristics. Some of these were:

- The tendency to overthink things.
- The tendency to entertain worst-case scenarios.
- The tendency to be responsible for too much.
- The tendency to be negative and pessimistic.
- And a big one – they all seemed to have an active and wild imagination.

If you are a victim of panic attacks, you can probably identify with some of these points. You probably don't like to admit it, but if you're honest with yourself, this is probably the way you're wired.

Learning to use my imagination for victory as opposed to bondage.

I quickly concluded that the imagination is very powerful. If my imagination had the ability to get me into trouble, then, with God's help, my imagination also had the ability to get me to freedom. I began to go on a campaign to reduce the vulnerabilities that the incorrect use of my imagination had created.

For a lot of you, you're going to just have to stop meditating on negative information, and you're going to have to stop letting a wild, unbridled imagination continuously take your thoughts to a place of entertaining doom and gloom. I believe you will find what is best for you by understanding what I did and adopting the same procedures, adding some little tweaks where needed. Whatever path is taken, there must be a reduction in speculation, and there must be limits on how and where negative thoughts can travel.

Continuing with my storyline, I learned to use my imagination in several helpful ways. I was out of the survival mode, but I wanted to learn to enjoy the ability to live in peace and in joy.

When you're dealing with panic attacks, it has the ability to make your mind very weak and tired. I didn't have the desire to physically go on vacations but I did have the desire to bless my mind with some peace and quiet. Amazingly, realizing the effectiveness of encouraging gymnasts to go through skills and routines in their mind because it increased their physical ability and skill was a technique I found beneficial for the help I needed.

I found naps to be helpful, but they did not stop my imagination from dwelling on possible negative scenarios. I began to intentionally use my imagination to dwell on positive scenarios. An amazing effective technique that I began to engage in was to go on vacations and visit places in my mind by way of my imagination.

Before you write me off, just remember that one of my strongest attributes is my logic. What I did was sit down in a quiet place and just allow my imagination to drift off and take me to some of my favorite places. No, let me correct that. In the beginning, I sat down and forced my imagination to take me to a good place.

My family had a cabin in the mountains, and before the onset of panic attacks, I would love spending time just sitting on the back porch overlooking the valley and the river. Amazingly, I found I had the ability to visit that exact place using my imagination. I would see myself sitting on the back porch and would create thoughts in my mind that supported what I would view as being very positive. Having always enjoyed wildlife, I would imagine seeing different animals in their natural habitat.

You must understand something; this was forcing me, the "All-American maintainer," to begin creating positive and carefree thoughts and thought patterns. *I was finally learning to entertain thoughts that I did not have to maintain.*

As I researched people who were inventors, I realized that what they invented had begun in their imagination. They could start with just an idea, which was born in their imagination, and end up with something grand. Take the airplane, for instance—how can something so heavy become airborne. Imagine that!

Without compromising my responsibility of maintaining the restaurants, I also began spending much more time imagining positive outcomes to different situations. I realized that it was a deception to think that I always had to speculate on the negative to be properly prepared to deal with it. My goodness, all the negative scenarios that I created over the years prepared me for a lifetime of readiness.

The more I correctly applied my imagination, the more I came to realize that my mind, and even my body, were beginning to benefit greatly from the activity that I was engaging in. Without realizing it, by meditating on the Word of God and through spending my time engaging in the use of my imagination to dwell on very enjoyable, positive scenarios, I found that my body was becoming much more relaxed and less susceptible to nerve sensitization. And get this: the more I pursued intentionally choosing my thoughts and what to meditate on, the more I found that *my body became much more resistant to the harmful release of adrenaline.* Talk about a breakthrough!

My thoughts were no longer forced to travel along a predetermined path at a high, uncontrollable speed, like our carefully iced sledding run. Even though, at this point in the storyline, I wasn't completely out of the woods concerning panic attacks, I found myself obtaining a type of mental freedom that I had not experienced since the onset of the first panic attack in 1992.

To recap what I began to adopt in my recovery process:

- Although I already somewhat restricted what I allowed my eyes and ears to be exposed to, I also chose not to watch or listen to daily news reports. I decided that if there was something earth-shattering that I needed to know or that I needed to pray about, I had plenty of people around me to keep me informed.
- I attempted to slow down any racing thoughts so that I could identify thoughts of speculation. I identified the thoughts of speculation and I verbally denounced them.
- And most significantly, I taught myself how to use my imagination to bring about peace of mind.

Please keep in mind that the things that I'm teaching you may seem unnecessary or even ridiculous to some people. Well, unfortunately, I wasn't "some people." I was a person who was susceptible to panic and anxiety attacks. As for you, you are reading this book to either obtain your own deliverance or to further educate yourself on how to assist other people in obtaining their freedom.

Allow me to finish up this chapter by giving you a few other tips that I found extremely helpful and which I used to obtain a strong healthy mind.

Sometime around 2001, I can remember how tired my mind was. To combat this mental fatigue, here are some of the things that I put into practice.

Reminders – One thing that I became aware of concerning the use of my mind was what I forced myself to remember. Because I was good at remembering, not only did I have my own dates and appointments to remember but my high level of dependability and self-driven level of responsibility would also often invite others to use me to remind them of things they did not want to forget. Therefore, I made some changes. I politely refused to take on the cares of others about the things that they really needed to be responsible for.

As for myself, I wanted to improve the quality of my sleep. As a very intentional process, before bed, I would sit down at my table and make a list of anything that was on my mind that needed to be resolved tomorrow or in the upcoming days.

I did my best to completely clear my mind of any possible weight. I would make notes and then intentionally attempt to forget about things. I worked to get to the point where I was surprised by the things on my list because I had chosen to clear my mind of things once I wrote them down.

With today's technology, you are blessed with the ability to set all kinds of reminders and to-do lists on your smartphone.

Back then, I was "rubbing two sticks together" and using Post-it Notes. Today, we have a BIC lighter and a smartphone. With these modern tools, you can sit back and clear your mind by making lists and setting reminders in a more efficient way.

Prioritize your time – your time is very valuable, and you probably have a lot to do. Therefore, it is important to learn to set priorities and make a list of what you feel you need to get done for the day. For myself, I would always make the list the night before.

Start with what must be done first—the most important thing on your list. Also, learn to tackle the things that you least desire to do—the things that you dread. Get them done and get them off your list. If you're going to have to do something by the end of the day, do it now. It's amazing how much better your day goes when you do not "drag dread" along with you all day.

Don't procrastinate – A lot of times people spend more time attempting to avoid things than the time it would take just to get them done.

Be good with your time. Learn to set a schedule that leaves you plenty of time so you do not feel pressure. Allow yourself ample time to arrive at scheduled destinations. Don't put stress on yourself by planning things too tightly.

If you often feel pressure to arrive places in a timely manner, or if you have a tendency for "road rage," leave a little extra time, anticipating that things are not going to go perfectly and that other people may not have the same priorities or the sense of urgency that you do.

Mistakes – Don't obsess about mistakes and failures. Failures are events, not people. Just because you fail at something, it does not make you a failure.

Maximize the use of your strengths and minimize the effects of your weaknesses. Don't beat yourself up—there are enough people in the world who are probably waiting in line to do that for you.

When you make a mistake or blunder, write down the mistake and then make a list of what you learned from it and what you plan on doing differently in the future. Then the most important thing: let it go and forgive yourself. If it comes up in your mind, just say out loud, "We have covered this. It is done, over, and I'm moving on." You may have to say that numerous times until you're finally able to let it go, but be persistent and resistant to torment.

Silence – I have observed that most people cannot handle silence. When there is silence, people become obsessed with the need to talk. Most of the time they have nothing to talk about, so they end up saying some of the most ignorant statements.

Learn how to handle silence. Learn how to lay your cell phone down and not check it constantly. Learn the blessing of being at peace and train your imagination to engage in good, healthy thoughts.

Arguments – Avoid arguments. Don't always feel that you must prove that you are right. Senseless arguments and debates can be very stressful. Even if you win the argument, what do you gain? A dog can usually always beat up a skunk, but is the outcome worth it?

God's Word – Learn to make time to meditate on the Word of God. Spending time in the book of Psalms and the book of Proverbs is a huge blessing to obtain peace of mind.

YOUR DEFENSE ARSENAL
"GO TO GUIDE"

There will be chapters of this book that you will want to continuously read over as a review, but within this chapter, I will provide specific directions on what to do in the onset of a panic attack and what to do in order to reduce the number of attacks, reduce the severity of attacks, and finally, end the attacks.

First and foremost, you must understand that I am not a licensed physician. Anything that you find in this book that opposes what licensed physicians have told you, their direction and instructions, should always supersede anything that I encourage you to do.

Second, as strongly as I can, I'm advising you to get a complete physical to obtain a clean bill of health. This is crucial to overcoming panic attack because you're going to have to learn to ignore some symptoms of your body that may appear to be frightening and significant. Firm evidence that you are in good health will enable you to more effectively ignore the symptoms obtained through speculation.

As I walk you through this chapter, I would like you to do your best to just relax and absorb the information. Trust me, we are going to begin to make a lot of progress toward putting an end to your panic attacks.

Also, be prepared to have some fun. In the beginning, I was so tense and uptight dealing with my panic attacks. However, I will show you how to get through this. If we learn how to avoid feeding into panic, the attacks will not last long. Meanwhile, you are establishing mental barriers and learning to look at life positively.

Remember the reason that I was so intentionally repetitive in my writing is so that the information will become ingrained within your thinking. By continuously feeding you the correct information, you have already begun to develop a new mindset, and you have already begun to develop helpful ways of thinking to establish correct thought patterns.

Through studying this book, up to this point, whether you realize it or not, we've started to minimize any negative mindset and any harmful patterns of thinking that you have allowed to be established within you. Understanding that, let's go on to obtain your victory. Relax, we're going to have a great time.

Vital point – the potential for panic attacks is not going to simply go away. On our path to recovery, you're going to experience the onset of panic attacks. I want you to be prepared so they do not catch you off guard and you do not experience any initial disappointment.

You are going to experience situations that are not dangerous, but they are still going to initiate uneasiness and fear within you. With the formation of fear, your body is going to release adrenaline into the bloodstream. That is what makes you feel very hyper and uncomfortable. The adrenaline is the cause of the racing heart, the difficulty breathing, and all the other symptoms that you experience.

Our initial attack is not to focus on trying to prevent the panic attack from ever happening; rather, our attack will be to first minimize the severity and the duration of the attack.

To obtain your freedom, you're going to have to learn how to control your reaction to what is happening.

The initial attack of panic will occur. Knowing that, I want you to be prepared to react properly. I want you to attempt to relax and understand that we fully expect this to happen.

What we're going to do first is to learn how to minimize our negative response to what you are experiencing.

First up, you have a little work to do. We're going to do some prep work and we're going to gather the supplies for your panic attack first aid kit.

Prep work:

1. Write down what you feel at the onset of a panic attack. For me, it was feeling of adrenaline surging through my body, a fast pounding heartbeat, and runaway thoughts. Write down what you have experienced in the past and up to this point.

2. *Your **emergency** statements of faith/truth.* Write down your relevant faith/truth statements. Compile a list and keep it with you constantly. I have included what I used at the end of this chapter for you to adopt, or you can write your own. Ideally, you should make a list of what you believe to be true. Up to this point, you have speculated on everything that could be wrong or go wrong. Now you're going to make a list of what you're going to choose to believe to be true over any feelings. This is to be used in an emergency. Either take a picture of my list and carry it with you, add to it, or make your own. Always keep a copy.

3. *A page or two of statements of faith/truth that you read daily.* Also, write out a more comprehensive second list of faith/ truth statements. Again, at the end of this chapter, I have included what I used for you to adopt, or you can write your own. You will read these statements daily. Initially, you will read them often, maybe once an hour. What we are doing is *intentionally interjecting what we choose to believe.* What you are doing is continuing to develop a new mindset and construct new thought patterns. Up to now, the thoughts that you have been entertaining have been somewhat

forced on you based on the way you feel. You are actually going to entertain thoughts that enable you to change the way you feel. When we feel differently, it becomes a lot easier to continue to think differently so that the thoughts that you choose line up with the behavior that you desire. Feelings are your emotions.

Emotions are powerful. Emotions are more powerful than logic. As we drive out speculation, you are going to begin to *choose how you want to feel.* How you feel will drive your thoughts. Initially, you are going to use thoughts to manipulate the way you feel. This sheet is going to be used daily.

4. *Compile some comedy to feed on.* This can be in the form of audio or video. For myself, I would go on YouTube and would set up a playlist for my smartphone. You can also download an app that allows you to have favored videos that you can pull up very quickly. This is something that you will want to continuously update so you have access to material that will have the most potential to be able to make you laugh.

5. *Begin to educate some go-to people.* Seek out people whom you trust and respect and who are reliable. You want them to be perceptive. You also want to have access to people who can make you laugh.

Some helpful tips:

1. Attempt to eat more frequent, smaller meals per day instead of just one or two large ones. When you feel bloated, it tends to make your normal breathing feel a little more restricted. Just as important, avoid going for a long time without eating to the point where you become very hungry. Hunger can cause you to feel anxious, which has the ability to bring about anxiety to initiate a panic attack. Learn to carry wholesome snacks with you, and it's a good idea to have access to water.

2. Do not consume candy or chocolate on an empty stomach.

3. Avoid caffeine.

4. It is very important to train yourself to breathe correctly. When we feel panic, we tend to breathe very quickly. Hyperventilation is a condition that occurs because of abnormally fast breathing. Healthy breathing occurs with a correct balance between breathing in oxygen and breathing out carbon dioxide.

Unfortunately, when we feel panic and anxiety, we tend to upset this healthy balance. There is often a rapid reduction of carbon dioxide in the body.

It is not necessary to know all the gritty details, but in essence, low carbon dioxide levels lead to a narrowing of the blood vessels that supply blood to the brain. This reduction in blood supply to the brain leads to symptoms like tingling in the fingers and toes and lightheadedness.

When you upset the healthy balance of breathing, you feel like you can't breathe or that you have to force yourself to breathe. Because of this, it's good to adopt the procedure of training yourself to breathe in through your nose for three seconds and then exhale through your mouth for three to six seconds. Along with this procedure, I have learned that, when I get my mind off of labored breathing, my breathing usually returns to normal. However, the discipline of breathing in and out correctly can be very important.

Procedures for the onset of a panic attack:

- If you feel the onset of a panic attack, take it as a challenge as opposed to a threat.
- Do not just sit around and dwell on how badly you feel. Do not strengthen harmful thoughts by meditating on them or entertaining them. You must reassure yourself that you are not in a life-threatening situation. You can handle this. Charlie the goat got out of the pen, but you are not going to feed him.
- If you feel like you are having trouble breathing, use the technique where you inhale for three seconds through your nose and then

exhale three to six seconds through your mouth. If you begin to feel tingly hold your breath for several seconds before you exhale

- Immediately go to your emergency list of statements of faith/truth. Speak the statements out loud even though you are most likely are not going to feel like doing this. In fact, I can almost guarantee that you are not going to feel like doing this, but force yourself to speak statements of faith and truth out loud. For myself, it would go something like this: "In the name of Jesus, I resist any fear and panic. Every organ and every tissue of my body functions perfectly. God is my Father, and I am protected from evil."

Force yourself to speak aloud and speak words of faith and truth that are in contrast to the way you feel.

If you are around other people, attempt to get your eyes off yourself and engage them in conversation even if it is people you do not know. You must force yourself to talk—to speak words—*OUT LOUD!* This is the fastest way to interrupt your negative thought pattern and to stop racing thoughts. Your mind isn't good at doing two things at once when the spoken word is brought into play.

You empower the thoughts by entertaining them. Speak words out loud that have nothing to do with the way you feel and speak words out loud that completely oppose the way you feel.

If you cannot think of any words to say, just start singing a familiar song with a positive message. Sing it out loud and boldly. Seeing as you want to go against the effects of adrenaline, a slower song is best, and be sure to concentrate on the lyrics. A simple example that everyone is familiar with would be the alphabet song. You can also add taking a slow deep breath every three to four letters to make sure you won't rush through it. Any song will get you thinking about something else. Make sure you keep a steady beat.

When you are successful in disrupting a harmful, fearful thought pattern, you will be successful in stopping the release of any further amounts of adrenaline into your bloodstream.

- Your first step is to attempt to handle it yourself using your words of faith/truth, the reason being that you always have this ability at your disposal. It is a great confidence builder to be able to stop the progression of a panic attack yourself. However, don't ever hesitate to use every weapon in your arsenal.
- If you are unsuccessful at stopping the progression of the onset of the panic attack, attempt to reach a friend by phone or go to them if they are at the same location that you are.

Initially, you will probably have to engage in negative thoughts and words as you let them know what's going on, but after that, attempt to restrict any negative thoughts or negative words. Eventually, you want to get to the point where you can call someone and just say, *"Help me."* This person should be prepared to help disrupt your pattern of harmful negative thoughts, just like I did with Maggie.

Engage them in conversation. Ask and answer questions. Initiate conversations that are totally unrelated to the way you are feeling.

When I was alone and I would reach out to a friend by phone, I would find it very helpful to have them on the phone while I read my daily sheet of statements of faith.

There were times where I would read this sheet up to five times before I felt the effects of the adrenaline that was released in my bloodstream begin to dissipate. After reading this book, it is important to keep fighting. Be confident that the attack will soon be over. You cannot stay in silence; you must speak words out loud.

- The other thing that I found for myself that was extremely helpful was to go to my supply of comedy videos.

You must either speak words out loud that oppose the way you are feeling or you need to be engaged in laughter.

If I felt the onset of a panic attack, I would often go immediately to my comical videos, and I would force *myself to laugh*. At the same time, I would comment on the video and say stupid stuff like, "That's funny. Check that out."

As you experience the onset of a panic attack, experiment with different ways to end it. I would go to videos where people were slipping and falling, just to enjoy stupid stuff. I would comment on what was going on and would force myself to get into laughter. When you become involved with something you are seeing AND hearing, it takes the focus off yourself.

I want you to experiment with this. You will have to learn what works best for you, but this is a very effective tactic.

Quick review: With the onset of a panic attack, our tactic is to do what it takes to end the duration of the attack as quickly as possible. Our efforts focus on the attempt to stop the release of any further adrenaline into the bloodstream.

- Don't remain idle.
- Breathe correctly.
- Force yourself to talk. Speak words of truth and faith or sing out loud.
- Engage people in a positive, distracting conversation.
- Call a friend for help.
- Watch comedy to initiate laughter. Find something that always makes you laugh.

Procedure for when the panic attack subsides and you regain control.

For some reason, adrenaline was released into your bloodstream without any apparent danger. Using the techniques previously listed, you have successfully stopped any further release of adrenaline into your bloodstream.

Immediately after the panic attack, there is always some cleanup work to do.

- Once again, it's important not to stay in silence. This is a perfect time for the art of speculation to kick in, and that's the last thing that we want, so we will not give it a chance. There will be a tendency to speculate on the speculation. Drop it. For the moment, forget it. It happened; you survived it. Do not hit the replay button. We are trying to erase the recording.
- Continue to read over your daily faith/truth statements. For myself, I would do this and then I would also begin to thank God for delivering me from the panic attack.
- When there are earthquakes in the natural world, they are always followed by aftershocks. When you have a panic attack, especially depending on the severity of it, there's also a tendency to have aftershocks.

Your body is in a heightened state of awareness. Your subconscious communicated to your body that there was danger present—even though there wasn't—but because the body perceived the presence of danger, adrenaline was released into the bloodstream by the adrenaline glands. After a panic attack, everything in your body tends to be a little bit on edge. We want to get to the place where we can relax. We want to make sure that the body does not continue to release small amounts of adrenaline into the bloodstream. Therefore, don't be alarmed by any little aftershocks. This is very normal, and handled correctly, it will not explode into another panic attack.

- Panic attacks can last anywhere from 10 to 30 minutes, with some even lasting up to an hour. This is unacceptable. If you handle things correctly, after the initial adrenaline rush, you will be able to get things back under control quickly using information that I've provided for you. The faster you stop the release of adrenaline, the faster the panic attack will come to an end. After that, your correct responses will minimize any potential repeat performances.

- Read the sheet of your statements of faith/truth. Have conversations with people. Watch or listen to some comedy. Do not just sit there and allow yourself to speculate on what just happened or what could possibly happen in the very near future. *It's over. Let it go.*
- It's very important to make sure that you are not entertaining negative, harmful thoughts. If you find that you tend to keep going back to negative thoughts, continue to engage in healthy conversation and read your statements of faith/truth out loud.
- After the panic attack, attempt to eat something light. Avoid spicy foods, avoid a lot of sugar, and definitely no caffeine.
- After a panic attack, you will usually feel a little tired. Position yourself where you can drift off to sleep while keeping your mind from entertaining negative thoughts. One option is to lie down and read a book out loud until you can just drift off to sleep.

Long-term maintenance

- It's very important to choose your words correctly. Learn to speak what you desire, not confirm situations in your life that you do not want.
- You must learn to create a new mindset, and you must learn to create new thought patterns. As you spend more and more time speaking words of faith and truth out loud, you will begin to create a new mindset, one that will help you minimize and eventually eliminate panic attacks.
- Continue to add more statements of truth/faith to your daily list. I like to refer to it as my confession sheet. What I'm doing is making confessions of the way that I choose to think. By deliberately choosing my thoughts and by meditating on them and speaking them out loud, I begin to change the way I feel.

The goal is to establish a new mindset and new thought patterns. With the correct mindset and with the correct pattern that your thoughts follow, it becomes more and more difficult for a potential panic attack to gain any momentum.

I do not speak
the way I feel.

I speak the way I want to feel.

I do not speak what I have. I speak
what I desire to have.

This is very important:

- You just don't get rid of a harmful mind pattern; you replace a harmful mind pattern with a healthy, desirable mind pattern.

  You cannot just stop thinking. Well, I take that back; I think I have witnessed some of my idiot friends possessing the ability to do just that. No, just kidding. Seriously, you just don't stop thoughts that you do not want; you learn to replace thoughts that you don't want with thoughts that you do want.

  This is why you must continuously meditate and speak desirable thoughts out loud. Use your **emergency** *faith/truth statements* at the onset of a panic attack but rely on your *daily statements of faith/ truth* to establish the correct mindset and thought patterns.

- A lot of people, through their struggle with panic attacks, have compiled a list of places or a list of things to do that they find to be unacceptable. In the previous chapters, I gave you several examples of situations and circumstances in my life that I found to be the initiators of fear, and therefore, I would avoid them. As you become stronger, you will be able to begin to go places and do things that, in the past, were not an option.

  Situations and circumstances that I am referring to are not anything that would normally be unsafe or risky.

I'm not referring to anything that people, in general, would describe as being daring. What I'm referring to are simple places—simple situations—that, for some reason, make you feel uncomfortable or stir up feelings of fear within.

Let's just say that it is very uncomfortable for you to go shopping in a certain large department store. As you get stronger, you begin to take back any ground, any territory that was taken from you by the threat of fear.

In a case like the large department store, you intentionally subject yourself to uncomfortable places to prove to your subconscious that they are not dangerous. Sometimes it helps to take another person along with you for the first time. You want to be prepared with your complete arsenal of weapons for defusing panic attacks. Each time you conquer what was previously deemed unacceptable, you become stronger and stronger at your ability to war against any future panic attacks.

Never put yourself in any danger. We are only subjecting ourselves to situations and activities that are not dangerous, but for some reason, your subconscious chose to label them threatening; therefore, we are proving our subconscious to be incorrect in its evaluation.

- Learn to reduce the stress in your life. Establish priorities that help you make good use of your time without feeling unnecessary pressure. Identify things that cause anxiety and do your best to reduce those things.

When you have dates and appointments, don't try to remember them. Make yourself notes and set reminders for yourself. It's amazing how many times self-induced anxiety has the ability to initiate a panic attack.

- Start intentionally, using your imagination to enable yourself to perceive situations from a positive view. Without realizing it, people are constantly using their imagination, but they fall into the rut of forecasting doom and gloom instead of learning how to anticipate a favorable outcome.

If you listen to people's conversations, most statements that people make involve a negative outcome. Remember, statistics show that 80% of a person's thoughts are negative. If your thoughts are negative, it stands to reason that your conversation will be negative.

People love self-pity. People love to draw attention to themselves. People seem to be in a competition to compete for who has the worst circumstances in their lives.

We must determine that this behavior is no longer an option. If you are going to put an end to the beast of panic attacks, you're going to have to be relentless in the way you think and speak.

As you intentionally choose your thoughts, you are going to develop a new mindset, and you are going to develop correct patterns of thinking. To do this, it is very effective to employ the use of your imagination. The imagination can be used to see a positive outcome for situations that you will be facing, and the imagination can be used to allow yourself to visit places in your mind—places that bring a very happy, content feeling.

When a person is engulfed in panic attacks, everything that goes to their imagination is initiated and driven by fear. As we learn to take control of our thought patterns, we are also going to learn how to direct our imagination to be able to choose to see positive outcomes to situations we face.

For myself, I had to intentionally choose the outcome that I wanted and then I would use my imagination to see that outcome. As I continued to do this over and over, it reinforced the new mindset that I was establishing, and I found that my thoughts were no longer driven to follow a harmful pattern.

In the past, the only thing that I could imagine was negative, undesirable outcomes. Today it is very hard for me to imagine anything negative. Please understand that I still maintain a high level of commitment to being responsible, but I refuse to meditate and speculate on potential negative outcomes that rarely ever actually occur.

Along with that, I use my imagination as a form of relaxation.

While I am in the process of going to sleep, I will imagine very positive situations instead of allowing my mind to over process the cares of the day.

Think of your mind as a movie screen and your imagination as the movie projector and film.

I can enjoy the mountains without ever leaving my house. I can enjoy the seashore and the ocean without having to fight traffic. If any of you find yourself feeling skeptical about what I'm telling you, just be very observant of how much you use your imagination in a negative way. For some reason, we are forced to conform in a world where anything negative is easily embraced, whereas anything positive is considered ridiculous. This negative imagination is common in those who worry have anxiety and in those that suffer from depression.

In high school, I used to do gymnastics, and while in college, I used to help coach and train gymnasts. Today I have a lot of fun seeing myself doing gymnastics skills in my imagination. Amazingly, what I enjoy in my imagination is far superior to anything that I was able to do through my own physical talents.

Well, I gave you a lot of suggestions for long-term maintenance. You will learn what works best for you. This chapter was devoted to preparing you to face panic attacks, survive them, overcome them, and learn to maintain your freedom from them.

Don't allow yourself to become disappointed or face discouragement. There is a time where I was not convinced that I would ever lead a normal life again.

I have defeated panic attacks in my life, and you will also defeat them in your life, too. You must be persistent; you must be diligent. You must be committed to knowing that you're going to win.

My statements of faith/truth.

As promised, I'm including what I used to fight off the onset of a panic attack and what I used to develop a new mindset and new thought patterns.

My statements of faith/truth, because of my belief in God and in Jesus Christ as Lord, are based on the promises of the Word of God.

Even if you do not have a firm relationship with God, one that is as strong as possible, I encourage you to adopt the statements of faith that I used. Press in and learn to trust God and rely on His promises.

I used this emergency list any time I felt the onset of a panic attack. I would speak them out loud to disrupt harmful thought patterns and runaway thoughts.

EMERGENCY FAITH/TRUTH STATEMENTS

- **In the name of Jesus, I take authority over any fear and panic.**
- **I resist fear and panic in the name of Jesus.**
- **I understand that I'm feeling the effects of adrenaline in my body. I am not in any danger. I demand that any further unnecessary release of adrenaline end immediately.**
- **I am in no danger.**
- **I am in perfect health**
- **I call these feelings of fear and anxiety to leave me immediately.**

I would continue to repeat these statements of faith/truth until I was convinced that the onset of fear was beginning to subside.

If you choose to use my list, I would strongly suggest that you add anything that you find to be helpful. With the onset of a panic attack, adrenaline has been released into your bloodstream by the adrenal glands. Your objective is to minimize your reaction to the adrenaline by refusing to enter into fear by entertaining harmful negative thoughts.

By successfully bringing an end to fear, you will ward off any additional releases of adrenaline into your body.

REVIEW YOUR STATEMENTS OF FAITH/TRUTH DAILY.

Our objective is to develop a new mindset so the way your future thoughts are processed are based on that new mindset.

Our objective is also to replace former negative thought patterns with new healthy thought patterns.

You will intentionally choose to meditate on thoughts that will ultimately determine how you think and how you feel. As you reconstruct the way you think and the way you feel, you will be able to gain control over how you behave.

Obtaining your objective of developing a new mindset and establishing new thought patterns will take diligence and persistence. Believe me, it is well worth the effort. This is what will maintain your freedom from being so vulnerable and susceptible to panic attacks.

It is crucial that you stop speaking negative and harmful words about yourself. The only time it is necessary to speak negatively is to briefly describe what is happening to your go-to person. This person should encourage you to just say, "Help me." However, from then on, you speak what you want, as opposed to what you are experiencing. This is a biblical principle that I will cover in future chapters. The Word of God says that *God calls things that are not as if they were.* In other words, God looks at the situation and doesn't confirm how it is; God confirms what He desires.

We are surrounded by facts. However, truth overrides and is superior to facts.

If you are experiencing something harmful, that is a fact. However, the Word of God is truth, which is superior to the fact of what you are experiencing. Therefore, as an act of your will, as a show of your faith, you speak words of truth to reveal what you believe the outcome will be, as opposed to simply confirming situations that revolve around the panic attacks.

I don't use my words to confirm harmful situations and circumstances; I use my words to change any harmful situation and circumstances. In *Mark 11:23*, the Word of God says that when a person comes to the place where they believe that what they say will come to pass, they will have whatever they say.

A lot of people say that's ridiculous. Those same people readily accept negative thoughts and speak negative words without being aware that this process brings about negative repercussions.

People invite tragedy and evil into their lives by continually speaking words that support the evil and the tragedy. People do not realize that they are the ones responsible for everything in their life that they wish was different.

A great example of this would be a person with depression and/or anxiety who goes to counseling for years. Every time, they dredge up the past, thereby bringing it to the forefront repeatedly. This repeated negative engagement has a stronghold on their lives; it BECOMES their life. These same people will regularly post on social media things about depression or anxiety, which only fortifies the problem. Many are of the mindset that if they keep facing the past, they will eventually be able to deal with it. However, you have to decide if you are going to live to maintain your life as is or fight to overcome what you remain hostage to. Unfortunately, people allow their circumstances to become their identity.

With this same person, when you ask them how they feel, seldom do you get the answer: "I feel great!" Somewhere in most conversations, they will go back to the past. This just reinforces the negative, which makes the ruts deeper and deeper. They want to be happy, but they have such deep ruts and runaway thoughts that they see no hope. They need to keep Charlie in the pen! But no one has ever shown them how.

We will soon be covering this in the next chapters. However, right now, I need you to be diligent to continuously speak words of faith out loud over your life. You are choosing to speak what you want, not what you have. By doing this, you will create a mindset that will support correct thinking. By thinking correctly, you'll replace harmful thought patterns with healthy, supportive thought patterns. The end result is that you will no longer be susceptible to the onset of a panic attack. This process will also be huge in helping people who struggle with uncontrollable levels of anxiety and any other mental torment.

This is the confession sheet that I used, but you can also create your own. If you choose to adopt it, continue to add to it so it is as effective as possible for you.

DAILY CONFESSION SHEET OF FAITH/TRUTH STATEMENTS

Jesus is Lord. Jesus is my Lord. Jesus is Lord over my spirit, soul, and body.

Jesus is Lord over any fear and panic. As an act of my will and a show of my faith, I resist fear and panic in the name of Jesus.

Panic attack—flee from me in the name of Jesus. The joy of the Lord is my strength, and the kindness and the covenant of peace from God will never depart from me.

My life is redeemed from destruction. Jesus has defeated the devil and all his works in my life.

No weapon formed against me shall prosper.

I am established in God's righteousness. Fear and panic will fall for my sake.

God executes righteousness and judgment for me against fear, oppression, and panic.

I am redeemed from the curse of the law, and I plead the blood of Jesus over my life.

I am the body of Christ. By the stripes of Jesus, I am healed.

Every organ and tissue of my body functions perfectly.

With a long life, my God will satisfy me and protect me from harm

I keep myself in the kingdom of light, love, and the Word, and Satan can't touch me.

I fear not, for God has given me the spirit of power, love, and sound mind.

God is on my side. Fear cannot operate in this body or mind.

I resist fear in the name of Jesus.

This sheet of confessions of faith was so crucial to both helping me through my survival mode and helping me establish the correct way of thinking.

I would read this sheet out loud at least twice a day. If I was at home and I got hit with a panic attack, I would immediately go to this sheet and read it out loud until I felt the fear and panic leave me.

I would force myself to concentrate on each statement as I read it out loud. I would also memorize it so that I could say it any time, wherever I was. I would often mix it up by reading it from bottom to top so that I had to concentrate on what I was speaking.

I believe I have supplied you with every tool that I used for overcoming and defeating panic attacks. As you press in to demand your freedom, I believe you will receive it.

I give God the credit and the glory for delivering me from panic attacks. God blessed me with wisdom and revelation knowledge on how to handle situations. The last chapters of this book will be dedicated to showing you the journey that I traveled to obtain the relationship with God my Father that I enjoy today.

Just as a lot of people struggle with panic attacks and anxiety disorder, many people struggle with their relationship with God. People are lost, confused, angry, skeptical, and complacent. So many people are getting beaten up by the world, and they have no idea how things will ever change. So many people are completely debilitated by addiction to drugs, alcohol, and other mental torments.

Through my journey to overcome panic attacks, I received the call on my life to minister to those who are being held hostage, not only to panic attacks, but to any form of evil in the world. I began my journey being very complacent, with very little trust. My life today— God has taught me truth and allowed me to see how His love for people destroys the work of the demonic realm.

FREEDOM FROM SPIRITUAL CONFUSION

THE "OTHER" JOURNEY

Well, what I just presented to you represented the build up to my first panic attack—that dreaded first episode, years of living in survival mode, years of learning to obtain my freedom, and finally, years of living out my freedom.

Yes, that was a wild ride. It was quite an experience. The only redeeming benefit is that everything I learned from being a victim of panic attacks carved a path that enabled me to quickly and effectively obtain my freedom.

When held hostage by my panic attacks, I so wished that I could get access to a book or information written by someone who had experienced panic attacks and who could show me the way out.

Without any doubt, I know that it was the will of God for me to write this book because God does not want people held hostage to a lifetime of fear and terror. Even more importantly, God does not want us to be ignorant, misinformed, or deceived in the revelation of the knowledge of Him. *Revelation Knowledge* means uncovering a deep understanding of God's truth.

I've just finished taking you on my journey to obtain freedom from panic attacks. Now I want to take you on one more journey—the journey that

I took to truly find God. If you do not believe in God or if you have not received Jesus as your Savior, this will be the most important journey of your life.

Years ago, when I was confused about God, I always wished that there was a simple book I could read that would tell me the truth about God. That way, I would be able to understand Him correctly. I tried to read the Bible, but I was never able to understand so many things. I always believed there was a God, but I also knew that at that time, I did not have a desire to seek Him, which left me in a very uncomfortable place to be.

Well, I finally found God, and He was not lost—I was! Now, covering the span of some 40 years, starting in 1979, I would like to take you on another journey to reveal to you what I was blessed to learn over the course of those years.

The title of this journey is "The Path." And specifically, I call it the path to *John 10:10.* In that Scripture, Jesus reveals that we have an enemy. The enemy comes to cause death, loss, and destruction. Jesus reveals that He came to bless us with abundant life.

If you do not know God, if you have no relationship with God, if you're confused about God, if you're angry with God, or if, up to this point, you had no interest in the whole subject, I only ask that you just open your heart and mind and allow God to speak to you through this story.

Trust me, it will not be boring, and it will not be condemnatory. By now, you know that I'm very logical and very driven. For me, to trust and believe in something is huge. I'm not flaky, nor am I manipulated by my emotions. I demand the truth and invest the time to obtain it. Along with that, once I obtain truth, I become committed to it.

Anyway, enough introduction. Let's get moving. Sit back, relax, and let your mind construct some new thought pathways. Join me on my "other" journey.

THE PATH

As a child growing up in the 1960s and 70s, I wasn't looking to stand out from the pack. In fact, I worked very hard just to blend in. Most of us lived in a way that we were seen and not heard.

At least, where I lived, things were very conservative. Most people attended church as a Sunday tradition, most people didn't view divorce as being an option, and very few of us were exposed to addictive drug use, which is prevalent today.

It was in my early childhood that God was pushed out of the classroom. We used to pledge allegiance to the flag, and we used to have a time of prayer. For the most part, we were very patriotic, and for the most part, the majority of us accepted the existence of God.

From elementary school through high school, nothing changed that much for me; in fact, nothing changed that much for many of us. Oh sure, there were a few rebels out there, but they were certainly in the minority.

As I discussed up to this point in my book, I was geared to live in safety and protect myself, and I was geared to encourage the safety and protection of others.

For me, the concept of God, or rather, the concept of a loving God, should have been just what the "doctor ordered." I mean, come on. What could be more important to a safety and protection guy like me than to believe in God—the God who offers eternal salvation?

Well, God wasn't important to me. I believed in God but had no desire to seek him. Actually, I would say that was common for most of my friends— the people I hung around with. We believed in God, and although we didn't challenge things, we just kind of went along with the flow.

As time went on, I realized that just acknowledging the existence, the presence of God was not enough for me. Too many things didn't make sense. There were too many things I couldn't wrap my mind around. Let me explain.

I tolerated church but did not necessarily enjoy it. I'm not isolating "church" to the point where we went as a family; it was any church that I visited or attended. For some reason, church just seemed like an extension of school—something you were just required to do whether you liked it or not.

For me, a person who was driven to know truth, there were some things that just didn't add up. Some of my confusion revolved around the following:

---

1. If God was God, why wasn't He part of our everyday lives?

If God was so omnipotent, where was He throughout the day? I mean, we honored God by going to church on Sunday, and we even got a "star" for our attendance in Sunday school.

My family participated in all the ceremonial rituals. For example, we prayed before we ate and we were expected to pray before we went to sleep (in theory).

My parents did an excellent job. They raised us correctly. However, they were just raising us the way they themselves were raised. God was for Sundays, mealtime, and bedtime prayer.

---

2. If God was a loving God, why would He teach people through pain and suffering?

Why did we refer to God as a loving God even though many believed He made bad things happen to us? I just couldn't wrap my mind around the way people made God responsible for everything bad that happened in the world. I would hear people say things like "Well, God made that person sick so He could teach them something. God allowed that family's house to burn down so they would appreciate what they had. God took that child so that the parents would rely more on Him."

You see, that kind of talk just didn't sit well with me. I had good parents. I had good grandparents. They didn't have to make me sick to get my attention. They did not have to destroy something of mine to make me appreciate what I had.

---

3. Why do people differ so much in what they believe
and what they do as far as a relationship with God?

I was raised in Lancaster County, Pennsylvania, which is well-
known for its Amish and Mennonite communities. There was
another stumbling block: what does choosing to live like
people who lived in the late 1800s have to do with pleasing
God? I highly respect the Amish and Mennonite communities.
They are extremely hard-working, but what would make them
think that God would be concerned about whether people
drove cars or not, or whether they had electricity or not?

But it was more than just the Amish and Mennonites.
Why were there so many different denominations?

4. Was God really in control of everything
that happened on Earth?

I was always told that God was in control. I was always
told that whatever happened was the will of God. That
kind of talk really put me in a tailspin. I mean, if God
was God and if He was in control, it just didn't seem
like He was doing a very good job at being God.

5. Why don't we see miracles today like were seen
in the days of the earthly ministry of Jesus?

Miracles were not only seen through Jesus; miracles were
also seen through the lives of people who believed in and
followed Jesus. Jesus spent two-thirds of His earthly ministry
healing people, raising the dead, and casting out demons.

As a kid and then as a young man finishing high school and college, questions like these never seemed to leave me.

It wasn't my intent to put the blame for my dilemma on other people. I just wanted to know the truth about who this God really was. If I'm going to believe in something, I want to know that I am committed to believing in the truth. If I am going to commit my eternal salvation to someone or something, I want to make sure that I am honoring the correct someone or something.

I can't say it was just the five points that I listed that I was struggling with; there were also other things.

I also pondered:

Why were there so many different denominations?

Why were there so many different religions?

Who was Jesus?

Who was this guy named Job?

I kept hearing about this Job guy who lived long ago. Why did God supposedly cause or allow many horrible things to happen to him? I needed answers.

Well, our timeline of these unanswered questions takes us to where I'd just graduated from college. No offense, but college only encouraged my confusion rather than helped clear anything up.

I remember how, for so many years, I would constantly ask God to help me understand the truth. I would continually pray just a very simple prayer: "God, I don't know you, I don't understand you, and I don't feel close to you—please help me."

Simple, but very honest and very direct.

After I graduated from college, I began to look for different career options in business. My parents owned a furniture store, so I worked there until I found what best suited me.

One day, a gentleman entered the store to buy some furniture. Somehow the conversation came up about how I'd just graduated from Penn State with a degree in food service and housing administration. The gentleman, Harold, complained about having problems in his restaurant, and he asked me if I wanted to help him out a little bit to get things under control. I gladly accepted the offer, and I began working for him part-time in the evenings and on the weekends.

It was a very nice operation, and the owners were good people. They seemed to be a little more outspoken about God and what they believed in than I was used to. So, I was very interested to see whether it was just talk or if they were prepared to back up the talk with the way they conducted their daily walk. There was some disparity. Nevertheless, at least I was being exposed to different aspects of God that I had never seen before. I started to wonder if this was God's way of beginning to answer my prayer to help me get to know Him better.

Within the business, there was a lady named Cindy who worked as a hostess for the restaurant. She told me that she and her husband were forming a Gospel group. While spending some time with Cindy and her husband, I found out that they were going through the same Christian growing pains that I was experiencing.

The influence of the owners of the restaurant had somewhat inspired me through their faith, but I knew there was a higher level, something more profound. Cindy, one or two other people, and I really shared a commitment to seeking God to gain revelation of His nature and His will for us.

As a group, we learned from different Gospel teachers to help us understand the Word of God correctly. As we strived to learn the Word of God, I started to gain an understanding. The information I was receiving was useful in helping me build a relationship with God. Thinking about reading the Bible may be overwhelming for many of you as it was for me. Listening to the Bible on CD is a very practical solution. Whenever I drove, I would listen to the Word of God.

From 1979 until 1981, I pressed on to seek and study the Word of God and continued to gain knowledge. At this point, it was still merely developing a deeper understanding, but at least it was something.

To help you follow the timeline, I worked with Harold for just a little while. In 1981, an opportunity presented itself for me to manage a new restaurant that was just being opened by Tom, the owner. This venture, over the course of a few years, grew to incorporate the five restaurants that I was managing when I experienced my first panic attack.

Jumping ahead, I continued to work for Tom until 2016 when two other employees and I were blessed with the opportunity to purchase the newest operation.

Allow me to give you a very quick overview of what I learned about God up to this point:

- ❖ God created the Earth. God created the Earth for mankind. The atmosphere of Heaven is spiritual, while the atmosphere of the Earth is physical.
- ❖ Because the Earth is physical, God created mankind with a physical body. He created the Garden of Eden, and He placed mankind—Adam and Eve—in the garden.
- ❖ Before God ever created the Earth and mankind, He ruled Heaven with three archangels: Michael, Gabriel, and Lucifer. Lucifer rebelled against God and was kicked out of Heaven. Lucifer deceived one-third of the angels in the rebellion, and they also were removed from Heaven.
- ❖ Lucifer was renamed Satan. Satan gained access to the Earth. Satan was no threat to God, so he set his sights on destroying mankind.
- ❖ Once Satan was removed from Heaven, he went from being spiritually alive to spiritually dead.
- ❖ Satan manipulated his way to gain access to Adam and Eve, and through deception, he was successful in deceiving Adam and Eve into disobeying God.

- When Adam and Eve disobeyed God, they were separated from Him. When they were separated from God, they were separated from the life of their creator.
- Every child born since the fall of mankind in the Garden of Eden has been born spiritually dead.
- Immediately after Adam and Eve disobeyed God and were separated from Him, He began to lay the groundworks to redeem mankind.
- For thousands of years, God began to make covenants with men and women on the Earth who would be obedient to Him. God was preparing the path for Jesus to be born.
- Jesus was born, matured, and began His earthly ministry at around 30 years old. Jesus taught mankind the truth about God, and He revealed the lies and deception of Satan—the enemy.
- Jesus lived a life of obedience, and He was crucified on the cross.
- Jesus gained access to the enemy and took back from the enemy what the enemy had received in the Garden of Eden through the deception of Adam and Eve.
- Jesus rose from the dead and is now seated in Heaven with God.
- Through Jesus, we are blessed to be able to once again regain our right standing with Father. Through Jesus, we are made righteous with Father. Through Jesus, we receive life, the eternal life that was lost in the Garden of Eden.
- When you receive life by being engrafted into Jesus, you will spend eternity in Heaven with Father.
- When we are made alive to God, we are empowered to be filled with the Holy Spirit—the Spirit of God.

Okay, I obtained information from the Bible, but what did all this really mean? It seemed to me that a lot of people accepted the information that I just listed for you, but I didn't really see it transform their lives. It's one thing to acknowledge something, and it's quite another to commit to believing in something.

To me, it was just information—just a story. I did not reject the information, but I certainly did not embrace this information as a life-changing revelation. I found myself accepting information, but obviously, there was a lot more to know. I realized that I was just like everyone else—I would say I believed in God, but I did not live out a lifestyle that was that much different from a person who did not believe in God. Wow, isn't that interesting? That was one of my main concerns – a very confusing point of how people can just acknowledge God without being transformed by their relationship with Him.

A lot of people say that faith is being able to believe what can't be proven. I say that true faith is the determination to overcome the impossible to prove that the Word of God is true.

Everything that I studied up to now provided me with theories, but I lacked verification. So, I set my sights on learning how to walk by faith. I still had those questions that needed to be answered.

Why isn't God displayed through a person's everyday life?

If God was a loving God, why would he teach people through pain and suffering?

Why are there so many denominations and so many religions?

Is God really in control of everything that happens on the Earth?

Why don't we see miracles today?

So, my journey continued. I had to figure out how the information that I had received up to this point would be able to take me to the revelation that I needed to have my questions answered.

I started out by listing information that I had recently acquired— information that I did not understand or embrace as I was growing up. Let me take that information and delve deeper into the specifics.

Lucifer, one of God's archangels, rebelled against God and was kicked out of Heaven. Somehow he ended up on the Earth.

Now, it stands to reason that if this Lucifer dude, now referred to as Satan, attempted to rebel against God and failed miserably, he had probably not finished in his attempts to cause problems. Obviously, Satan was in no position to harm God. It started to become apparent that God intentionally created man and woman so that He could have a relationship with them. *Well, it stands to reason that if Satan could not attack God, he would set his sights on attacking what God loves.* That's us. Okay, that's a big point. I don't know why God didn't destroy Lucifer, but obviously, for whatever reason, He did not, so Lucifer, now referred to as Satan, would still need to be dealt with.

Revelation – We have an enemy.

****

What responsibility do we have if this whole God thing is true? Do we just sit around and wait for this Satan dude to move in and beat the pulp out of us? It says that God created the Earth, all the animals, and then He made man. So, He must have expected us to have some responsibilities, just as any parent would. Time to find out what responsibility God gave to man through His word.

> **Genesis 1:26 – 28 (AMP): God said, Let Us [Father, Son, and Holy Spirit] make mankind in Our image, after Our likeness, and let them have complete authority over the fish of the sea, the birds of the air, the [tame] beasts, and over all of the earth, and over everything that creeps upon the earth. 27 So God created man in His own image, in the image and likeness of God He created him; male and female He created them. 28 And God blessed them and said to them, Be fruitful, multiply, and fill the earth, and subdue it [using all its vast resources in the service of God and man]; and have dominion over the fish of the sea, the birds of the air, and over every living creature that moves upon the earth.**

Whoa, I thought, *this is a game changer.* Here's what I received:

God made mankind in His image and His likeness.

Why would He do that? It had to be for the purpose of a relationship. Wow, check this out: mankind—men and women—was given the responsibility, the authority over what happens on the Earth.

No one had ever taught me that.

Revelation—We were made in the image and likeness of God, and we were given responsibility for what happens on the Earth.

****

God gave Adam and Eve strict instructions to walk in authority. God also gave them one restriction: there was a tree present in the Garden of Eden, the tree of the knowledge of good and evil, and they were not allowed to eat from that tree.

As the story goes, the enemy, Satan, approached Eve and deceived her into eating the fruit that they were not supposed to eat. Adam messed up because he did not take authority and drive the enemy out of the garden; instead, he ate the forbidden fruit as well.

Because they both ate from the tree of the knowledge of good and evil, thereby disobeying God, they separated themselves from the life of God, and the power and authority that were once in their possession were now given to the enemy.

Through deception, mankind disobeyed God and thus became separated from Him. Satan received the power and authority that had once belonged to mankind. This is confirmed in the book of Luke when Satan tempts Jesus in the wilderness. The only power that Satan has is limited to being able to deceive people.

> **Luke 4:5 – 6 (AMP):** Then the devil took Jesus up to a high mountain and showed Him all the kingdoms of the habitable world in a moment of time [in the twinkling of an eye]. 6 And he said to Him, To You I will give all this power and authority and their glory (all their magnificence, excellence, preeminence, dignity, and grace), for it has been turned over to me, and I give it to whomever I will.

Revelation – The enemy deceived Adam and Eve into disobeying God. The repercussions of the disobedience caused Adam and Eve to be separated from God, and Satan received the power and authority that mankind was to walk in. We have an enemy, and the enemy works by deception.

****

What I was learning was really cool. Through the new information that I was taught by different teachers, the Word of God gave me confirmation.

You must understand that, at this point, I merely had a lot of information. The stories and information were great, but how do I know that they were true? If I were to share this information with others, what would compel them to believe me? I needed something to offer them that would bring about *verification* that what I was sharing was correct. If the information was "truth," then following that truth would have to have the ability to empower me to live differently than someone who does not believe in God and walk out the truth.

At this point, my new information:

- We were created in the image and likeness of God for the purpose of a relationship.
- We were given authority over Earth.
- We have an enemy—Satan—who works through deception. When Lucifer, now Satan, rebelled against God, Satan deceived

one-third of the angelic realm to follow him. This is now known as the demonic realm.

- Satan tricked humankind into disobeying God. Through this deception, mankind bowed their knee to Satan. Since God gave everything to humankind and then, through deception, humankind gave everything to Satan, this positioned Satan to become the god of this Earth and the god over fallen mankind.

At this point, my new information brought about some possibilities that would clear up things that never made sense to me before. I started asking myself questions. The answers to these questions built the solid foundation upon which I now stand.

Could it be that, due to an enemy who works through deception, people were deceived as to who they are called to be and the responsibility that they are called to carry?

Could it be that the evil that occurs on the Earth is not from God but rather the result of the influence of the demonic realm?

Could it be that people, in their efforts to honor God and to remain humble, walk *away from their responsibility* and then declare that God is in control and whatever happens on the Earth is the will of God?

Could it be that the enemy works very hard to cause death, loss, and destruction as an effort to hurt God by having Him watch mankind being destroyed?

Could it be that, through deception, we further disappoint God by blaming all the evil that the enemy causes to actually be the works and the will of God?

Could it be that, through the disobedience of Adam and Eve, Satan gained ownership of the earth and control over mankind?

Could it be that the reason that God did not destroy Satan was that, if God destroyed him, it would then have caused the destruction of the Earth and, even more importantly, the destruction of humankind?

Could it be that God loved humankind so much that He was willing to send His son Jesus to redeem humankind and take back what was lost in the fall of humankind in the Garden of Eden?

Could it be that God's love for us is more powerful than we ever imagined? After all, God made us in His own image. God refers to Himself as our Father, and He also refers to us as His sons and daughters.

At this point in the timeline, we are working our way through the 1980s. I had always wanted to believe in God, but now I found myself being more motivated to seek the truth to position myself to know Him better. My foundation was built on the following:

1. God created Heaven and Earth, and God created humankind so that we could have a relationship with Him. God refers to Himself as our Father.
2. God gave the responsibility of the Earth to humankind; however, humankind messed up and allowed it to be transferred to the demonic realm.
3. God sent His son Jesus to undo the works of the enemy. Jesus took back what humankind lost to Satan. Jesus died for us so that we could be forgiven for our sins. He also died for us so that we could be made alive and put back in right standing with God.

I had a foundation, but my foundation was still weak. Not only did I want verification for my foundation, I wanted it to be strong enough to commit my life to.

As I continued to study, I came across a story in the Bible that was pivotal for me. The story takes place during the time of the earthly ministry of Jesus.

> Mark 4:35 – 41 (NKJV): On the same day, when evening had come, Jesus said to His disciples, "Let us cross over to the other side." 36 Now when they had left the multitude, they took Him along in the boat as He was. And other little boats were also with Him. 37 And a great windstorm arose, and the waves beat into the boat, so that it was already filling. 38 But He was in the stern, asleep on a pillow. And they awoke Him and said to Him, "Teacher, do You not care that we are perishing?" 39 Then He arose and rebuked the wind, and said to the sea, "Peace, be still!" And the wind ceased and there was a great calm. 40 But He said to them, "Why are you so fearful? How is it that you have no faith?" 41 And they feared exceedingly, and said to one another, "Who can this be, that even the wind and the sea obey Him!"

This simple story opened up so many potential truths. It also helped me overcome much of the confusion that I was experiencing.

- Jesus was crossing the lake with His disciples, and a huge storm hit.
- The storm was obviously not caused by God, because Jesus rebuked the storm. The thought of Jesus rebuking God would be preposterous.
- Jesus didn't pray; He simply spoke to the storm, saying what He desired to happen.
- The storm was obedient to the words of Jesus.
- Jesus rebuked the disciples for their lack of faith.

This put me on a wild journey to study the ministry of Jesus. In *John 14:9,* one of the disciples asked Jesus to reveal God to him. In response, He made an astounding statement:

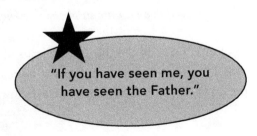

"If you have seen me, you have seen the Father."

Why had I never been taught this before? This changed everything. This cleared up so much deception, which I was quickly coming to realize needed to be attributed to the demonic realm. As I studied the earthly ministry of Jesus, this is what I found:

- Jesus never refused to heal anyone.
- Jesus never told anyone that their sickness was from God and that God was trying to teach them something through that sickness.
- Jesus rebuked any storm he encountered. Jesus never blessed a storm and sent it to destroy towns or cities so they could come to know God better.
- Jesus revealed that we have an enemy and that the enemy comes to steal, kill, and destroy.
- Jesus revealed that He came to bless people with abundant life.
- Jesus revealed that He came to undo and to destroy the works of the enemy.

Then I came across one of Jesus's promises that changed my life.

> **John 14:12 – 14 (NKJV): "Most assuredly, I say to you, he who believes in Me, the works that I do he will do also; and greater works than these he will do, because I go to My Father. 13 And whatever you ask in My name, that I will do, that the Father may be glorified in the Son. 14 If you ask anything in My name, I will do it."**

Again, why was I never taught this in the past? As I meditated on the question, the answer was obvious.

The works that Jesus did—the miracles, signs, and wonders—were works that could not be done through a man's own human physical strength.

The only way that a human can do the things that Jesus did is if they are empowered by God. Therefore, if someone does the impossible, that is a verification that proves that God is God. Look at the following Scripture:

> John 10:37 – 38 (AMP): If I am not doing the works [performing the deeds] of My Father, then do not believe Me [do not adhere to Me and trust Me and rely on Me]. 38 But if I do them, even though you do not believe Me or have faith in Me, [at least] believe the works and have faith in what I do, in order that you may know and understand [clearly] that the Father is in Me, and I am in the Father [One with Him].

That is absolutely astounding. Basically, Jesus is saying, "If I do not do the works of My Father, works that are impossible through My own human physical strength, then you are off the hook; you do not have to believe Me."

This is a challenge that Jesus presented to the people during His earthly ministry who did not believe that He was the son of God.

Well, if you followed that truth, then I realized that I should make the same statement to prove that God is the one true God. Jesus was able to do the miraculous because He is the Son of God. Those people were present to see Jesus do the impossible. But then Jesus goes on to say that, if a person truly believes in Him, they will thus be empowered to do the same works that He did.

If I walk out or experience a lifestyle that is impossible to live through my own human strength and effort, then everything that I learned about God just went from being a theory to being the undeniable, indisputable truth!

Let's do a quick review:

- ✓ God had three archangels. One of them, Lucifer, attempted to rebel against Him. Lucifer, renamed Satan, was kicked out of Heaven and took one-third of the angelic realm with him.
- ✓ God created the Earth. God created the Earth for mankind. Earth was a physical expression of Heaven. God made men and women after His likeness in His image. God created mankind

for relationship. God chose to refer to Himself as Father and to humankind as His sons and daughters.

✓ God would enjoy a relationship with His children as they followed out the responsibility to have charge over the Earth. His children were alive physically and spiritually.

✓ Satan, in an effort to attack God, found his way onto the Earth, entered the body of a snake, and proceeded to deceive Eve and manipulate Adam so that they would disobey their Father.

✓ In their disobedience, they lost their relationship with God as their Father and were reduced to being alive physically but not spiritually, and they lost the power and authority that God gave them to run the Earth.

✓ God could have destroyed Satan at this point, but that would mean He would also destroy the Earth and mankind because they were now under Satan's authority.

✓ God immediately began to form relationships with men on the Earth, men like Abraham, Noah, Moses, and many more to begin to get access back into the Earth.

✓ This is huge, and you will have to listen carefully. God is almighty, God is sovereign—God is God. He can do whatever He wants— everything except *lie* and *violate who He is*.

As an act of the will of God, He created the Earth, and He gave the responsibility for the Earth to mankind. God gave the responsibility of the Earth to mankind with a full understanding that this could cause Him to be vulnerable to what He created.

God equipped humankind with the freedom to make their own decisions and actually speak their own chosen words. None of the angels had the freedom to do this.

✓ Because God gave humankind access to the Earth and mankind was deceived by the demonic realm to disobey God, the door was open for the demonic realm to hold power and authority on Earth.

- ✓ Remember, God was fully able to step in and destroy Satan, but His creation and mankind would have been destroyed along with him.
- ✓ As I said, to gain access back into the Earth, God began to make covenant relationships with men who were willing to follow Him.
- ✓ The objective of God was to begin to get His Word into the Earth to pave the way for His Son Jesus to be born into the Earth to redeem humankind from the demonic realm.
- ✓ God spoke His Word into the womb of Mary, who then conceived Jesus. It had to be a virgin birth because of the curse that came upon the bloodline of humankind after the fall of Adam and Eve in the Garden of Eden. Hence, Jesus had to have a pure bloodline that was not cursed.
- ✓ Jesus was born, and at the age of around 30, He was baptized in water. When he came out of the water, the Spirit of God descended upon Jesus and filled Him. Before this, Jesus lived simply as a normal boy growing into manhood. He needed to experience everything we would go through in life. This is why Scripture states—He grew in favor with God and with Man.
- ✓ When God made Adam, He breathed His spirit into Adam. Humankind was filled with the life of God. In the fall of humankind in the Garden of Eden, humankind took on the nature of Satan, which was to be dead spiritually because Satan was separated from God.
- ✓ For the first time since Adam and Eve, a man—Jesus—was once again filled with the life of God. Please understand that Jesus was God's (only begotten) Son. However, Jesus laid aside His divinity, took on flesh, and walked the Earth as a man (*Philippians 2:7 – 8*).
- ✓ God gave the authority of the Earth to mankind, and mankind disobeyed God and caused the authority to be given to Satan. *This is huge—a man, Adam, gave the authority away. Then Jesus, now born a man, filled with the Holy Spirit, would be empowered to take back what Satan had stolen from mankind.*
- ✓ It's very interesting to see that Satan was only mentioned a few times in the Old Testament. As soon as Jesus was filled with the Holy Spirit, Satan and the demonic realm were exposed. For the

first time since Adam and Eve, a man on the Earth was made alive and filled with the Spirit of God, and He would have the power and authority to control the demonic realm.

✓ Throughout the earthly ministry of Jesus, He healed everyone who came to Him to be healed. *Why? Because Jesus was filled with God and sickness and disease is not of God.* Jesus also continuously drove out demons who were harassing people. Why? Because Jesus was filled with the presence of God. The presence of God drives out the demonic realm.

✓ Jesus was obedient to death and allowed Himself to be crucified.

✓ When Jesus died, the demonic realm thought that they had succeeded in destroying Him. However, because Jesus never sinned and because He had the eternal bloodline of God, He was able once again to be filled with the Holy Spirit and raised from the dead. During that transformation from death to life, Jesus defeated the enemy and took back the authority that had been lost in the Garden of Eden. This is recorded at the end of the book of Matthew, where Jesus says, *"All authority has been given to me, both in Heaven and on Earth."*

✓ Jesus ascended to Heaven and was glorified. When we choose to receive Jesus, the Word of God says that we become engrafted into Him. Our spirit can once again be made alive to God—that's why Jesus referred to the transformation as being "born again."

✓ When a person is made alive to God, they are then blessed with the amazing privilege of being able to be filled with the Holy Spirit—the Spirit of God.

✓ When people are made alive to God and filled with the Holy Spirit, they are empowered to take their places as sons and daughters of Father, and they are empowered to undo the works of the enemy just as Jesus did.

Okay, as we follow the timeline of working through the 1980's, just rounding the corner into the 90's, I had begun to build quite an arsenal of information from the Word of God that began to offer potential answers to a lot of my questions:

Why wasn't God active in the everyday life of people who said they believe in Him?

I must answer this by saying that I don't believe that most people who say they are Christians have been taught the truth. There is a big difference between acknowledging God and actually believing in God. Without the truth, many accept that going to church and saying an occasional prayer are what God is all about. When truth is taught, we, as sons and daughters, understand we are to seek a relationship with Father.

Why is God blamed for bringing harm and sickness to people?

Wow, I could write a book on this one. Sorry, I guess I am writing a book. Anyway, this question really needs to be cleared up. I have included a few revelations below:

- We have an enemy. There is a demonic realm that opposes what we are to accomplish.
- Throughout the Old Testament, humankind was not equipped to deal with the demonic realm because it could not be filled with the Holy Spirit.
- God did not mention the demonic realm very much in the Old Testament for that very fact. Because of that, God took the blame for all the evil that occurred.
- Then Jesus came to reveal the Father. Do people understand this? If people understood this, then maybe they would not blame God for everything evil that happens. Again, as I study the ministry of Jesus, I do not see where Jesus blessed any sickness or blessed any tragic circumstances.
- God is not the one who brings about damnation. The enemy causes damnation. That's why associating damnation with the name of God is to take the name of God in vain. As a side note, do you understand that, if you associate damnation with the name

of God, you are thus referring to Satan as your god? That'll give you something to think about.

- Do people actually understand that God gave humankind the responsibility for what goes on here on the Earth? Obviously not!

Everything that happens on Earth is not the will of God. If it was, then Jesus would never have had to intervene to make corrections.

- People often say that God is in control. I disagree. God is in charge, God is almighty, and God is sovereign, and within His sovereignty, He chose to make humankind responsible for what occurs on the Earth. I will cover this later, but basically, God is always in charge and the only time God is in control is when humankind chooses to develop a relationship with God and we take the responsibility to carry out His will.

Again, so much information. It's starting to make more sense; things are starting to come together, but it still remains just a theory. How do we bring verification of the theory to be able to deem it as truth?

Well, in the earthly ministry of Jesus, He gave me the path to verification.

Jesus told us that He perfectly revealed the Father.

> **Jesus** told the people who were present during his earthly ministry that the works that He does reveal the truth about God.

> > **Jesus** said that the person who believes in Him will be empowered to do the same works that He did.

As I began to meditate on all the information that I had compiled, there was one way to take this information, which remained in the form of a theory, to a place where it would be verified as truth. That one way would be to walk in the ability to minister to people as Jesus did, where power and authority were released through my life because of my commitment to believe in and have faith in God.

Please understand that, by this time in my life, verification or no verification, I chose to fully believe in God.

I believed in God. I received Jesus as my Savior, as the Lord of my life, and I pressed in to learn more and more about what I had access to concerning the promise of being able to be filled with the Holy Spirit, the Spirit of God.

As I began to put my trust in God and His word, my faith began to grow. God blessed me with the ability to effectively witness to people to tell people what I had learned about God.

I also began to pray for people. Most of my prayers were for people I knew. I would pray that they would trust God and receive their salvation by accepting Jesus as Lord. Also, I began to pray for simple ailments, such as headaches, to be gone and other things like that, but nothing that would be considered an indisputable miracle.

At this point in the book, we are approaching 1992—the year that I experienced my first panic attack. The gentleman that I worked for at the time, Tom, had just acquired a large restaurant—around 600 to 700 seats, a 60-room motel, and extensive gift shop. Just to help you clarify things, this eventually became the facility that my two partners and I purchased in 2016.

At this point, I was responsible for overseeing four other restaurants that Tom owned. Now it was also my responsibility to oversee this large facility that he had just purchased.

Anyway, I have a very interesting story to tell you that occurred in 1992, just before my first panic attack. I'm looking forward to telling you about it, and we will pick up on that story in the next chapter.

A MAJOR BUMP IN THE ROAD

Our timeline begins in the early months of 1992. The gentleman I worked for, Tom, had just purchased a new restaurant.

In the past, my job was probably the most important thing in my life. A shift had definitely been taking place to where I now put the desire for my relationship with God above everything else. I was on a journey—I was on a mission. I was determined to walk out the Gospel of Jesus Christ in truth.

My questions about God were finally beginning to be answered. In the past, I always questioned why God wasn't a huge part of a person's everyday life. I started realizing that God was not central to the lives of most people because they did not invite God to be the core of their life. They were compromising to add something new instead of committing to God and His Word to become something new. As the Scriptures say, "Draw near to God, and God will draw near to you." Well to me, people were drawing near to everything except God.

I questioned why God was always blamed for the evil that happened. Again, I found the answer to be in the Scriptures. Jesus came to truly reveal the nature of God. Instead of committing to press in to learn the truth, people were more comfortable being taught tradition instead of the authentic Gospel. Jesus made it clear that we have an enemy who comes to steal, kill, and destroy. Jesus came to bless us with abundant life. Hence, we need to press into the Word of God and allow the Holy Spirit to reveal the true nature of God.

I have questioned why people always say that everything that happens is the will of God. In conclusion, I decided that it isn't. If it was, Jesus would not have healed the sick and raised the dead. Jesus revealed the nature of my Father. The enemy is a liar and operates through deception. You can't allow yourself to be exposed to incorrect teaching. Jesus said that you are filled with the Holy Spirit and the Holy Spirit will take you to all truth.

I questioned why there are so many different denominations. Again, it is because we do not walk out the Gospel in power and authority to reveal the authentic Gospel. Compromise will always bring about counterfeit. Walk out the authentic, and the counterfeit will not have an opportunity to emerge. Unless darkness sees the true light, it will always assume that it is light itself.

People have been deceived into conforming to this world. People have not pressed into the Word of God to experience a transformation of the renewing of their mind. The degree to which I can renew my mind to the Kingdom of God is the degree to which I can experience Heaven while I am on this Earth.

Jesus said that He is the head of the Church and we are the body. There cannot be multiple bodies—multiple denominations. The only way to have multiple denominations is to have multiple heads of the church. There is only one head of the Church, and that is the Lord Jesus Christ. Pastors must be committed to preaching Jesus, to gathering people to Jesus, and not preach their own personal agenda.

Victory is the affirmation of trusting and believing in the one true God. Compromise is the interjection of human logic and reasoning to lower the definition of victory to enable us to still feel good about ourselves in the midst of defeat. Furthermore, people give mental assent instead of spiritual commitment, and the end result is a lifestyle of the Church that does not stand out from the lifestyle of the world.

Okay, Brian, calm down. There'll be plenty of time to preach later. As you can tell, by pressing into the Word of God, I began to be very passionate about what I believed. Could it be that my passion for God positioned me to be a target for the demonic realm? Let's continue the journey.

The opening of a new restaurant, or the taking over of an existing restaurant, had become pretty much routine for me. I had four under my belt, and the present would be the fifth operation.

I guess the difference with this operation was mainly the size of the facility. Most of the other restaurants only seated around 200 people, whereas this facility could seat between 600 and 700 people. Along with that, this facility had a 60-room motel, and up to this point, while I had been trained to run a motel, I'd never had the opportunity to acquire hands-on experience.

As an owner, Tom did not have much desire to be involved in the day-to-day operation of the facilities that he owned. He pretty much put me in charge of overseeing the operations, and I would meet with him once or twice a week to give him an update on how things were going.

Tom had purchased this most recent restaurant and motel facility from his friend Ed. Ed was a great guy, but he was ready to retire and was very glad to be able to sell the facility that he owned to his friend.

Since this facility was well-established, I basically just had to go in and oversee the management staff that was already in place. I would always try to work with the management team as opposed to just cleaning the house and starting over.

Over the last few years before I was brought into the picture, Ed had not kept a very close eye on his facility, and a lot of the employees were a little too carefree. I felt I had to instill a new sense of accountability within the employees and the management team. It was up to me to install systems that would benefit both the facility and the employees.

DEMONS IN THE DUNGEON

Kids will be kids, and employees will be employees, but I came across a situation that was definitely unique and outside of any norm that I had ever experienced. With my typical perceptive and watchful eye, I began to notice some unusual behavior among some of the employees. Keeping a close ear, I began to hear talk about how some of the young employees, who were in their teens and early 20s, would sneak back into the restaurant at night and hang out in a very secluded room under the restaurant. It was an unfinished part of the basement where the water pumps, water softeners, and equipment like that were located.

Through further investigation, I was shocked—no, let's change that to horrified—to find out that these young employees were sneaking back in at night to have séances and demonic worship. I had never been exposed to nor ventured anywhere near that basement area. I thought it was high time to examine exactly what we had going on. By the way, I chose the daytime hours to do my examination—my mother did not raise a fool!

This room was dark and dingy. It had a crushed stone floor with poor drainage so that the air was very humid. However, it was more than just humid—the atmosphere seemed to be thick, almost tangible. I sensed a type of weightiness that came on me, as well a type of restriction as I endeavored to move about the room. Since then, I have found out that others who have entered places of demonic worship also felt this same unusual weightiness.

As I cautiously began my exploration, I ventured into the restaurant dungeon with substantial uneasiness. Sure enough, I found a circle made up of a creative selection of seats most likely acquired from rummaging through garbage dumpsters. In the center of the circle was a fire pit where they burned incense and who knows what else! There was what appeared to be demonic symbols on the walls with a lot of skull-and-crossbones artistry thrown in for good measure. What appeared to be blood, but which was most likely touch-up paint from the maintenance room, was smeared upon the walls in efforts to obtain whatever ambiance that they were going for.

As I made an even closer inspection, I concluded that, in some areas, there was actual blood, which had been used to provide parameters in which the demonic worship supposedly took place.

Well, I had seen enough. Whatever was going on in that well-crafted demonic hangout, I wanted nothing to do with, and I certainly did not want to allow it to continue within the restaurant facility that I was responsible for.

Having pressed in to learn a lot about God and the earthly ministry of Jesus, I was very aware that Jesus spent a good portion of his time driving out demons. I knew it must be the right thing to do but knew very little about it.

I gathered up the employees responsible for this little Den of Horrors and attempted to explain to them that what they were messing around with was so much more serious and harmful than they could ever imagine. As I educated the misguided night owls, they began to understand the gravity of what they were choosing to play around with. After educating the employees on how the demonic realm works through deception to cause people to open the door to death, loss, and destruction, they seemed well motivated to put an end to what they mistakenly viewed as harmless fun. They had no foundation in good versus evil, and thus, they were easily manipulated.

It didn't take long before the dungeon was transformed into a clean, well-lit room devoid of blood/paint, demonic pictures, and a variety of skulls and crossbones.

Amazingly, the atmosphere in the room became so much lighter and so much less constrictive. Everything was cleaned up, and we were back on track. At least, that's what I thought.

You can take this for what it's worth, but within three to six weeks after I shut down the demonic dive, I became terrorized by my first panic attack.

Having said that, let me immediately put out a few disclaimers:

- I don't necessarily believe that everyone who suffers from panic attacks or anxiety disorder is dealing with demonic oppression.
- Anyone who is born again and filled with the Holy Spirit has the power and authority to cast out demon spirits.
- The demonic realm works through deception. The demonic realm must deceive mankind to be vessels through which demonic activities can be accomplished.

After everything I now know, let me give you my take on the situation.

With everything that I just explained to you in the previous chapters, I believe that I opened myself up to be vulnerable to panic attacks and anxiety attacks through being overly watchful with a tendency to overthink and overanalyze.

I had a mindset that invited harmful thought patterns based on the use of speculation.

With all my vulnerabilities in place, I believe I opened the door for demonic oppression to move in and give me the push that I needed to start the process rolling to be entrenched in debilitating panic attacks. Amazingly, it was not until years down the road that I received the revelation of how I opened up the door to set myself up for demonic oppression.

As I pressed in to learn from the Word of God and in the years that followed my first panic attack, I began to gain a greater insight into the spiritual warfare that takes place between the kingdom of light and the kingdom of darkness.

One other thing that must be discussed is the focus the demonic realm has on potential opposition. In *1 John 3:8* (NKJV), the Word of God says, *"For this purpose, the son of God was manifested, that He might destroy the works of the devil."*

Jesus was a threat to the demonic realm. I believe the demonic realm worked through the Pharisees and other religious leaders during the earthly ministry of Jesus in an attempt to keep Him from walking in power and authority to undo the works of the enemy.

I believe that anyone who is committed to waging spiritual warfare against the kingdom of darkness will show up on their radar as a potential threat.

We are filled with the Holy Spirit and the presence of God. The demonic realm is no match for us because greater is He who is in me than he that is in the world. The Word of God says that when we resist the enemy, the enemy flees in terror. However, it is very important to be well grounded in the Word of God and to be prepared to stand your ground against any demonic attack.

I believe I was getting to the point where the demonic realm could possibly look at me as a threat. Not on my own strength and ability, but because I was obediently yielding to be filled and empowered by the Holy Spirit.

If I had known in 1992 what I know today about panic attacks, I believe the duration of the affliction would have been extremely short. If I had known in 1992 what I know today about spiritual warfare, I believe I would have been prepared to put a stop to any demonic oppression before it had an opportunity to start.

From 1992 until 2004, I had a lot of years to devote to learning more about my Father— God—as well as Jesus my Savior and the amazing privilege to be filled with the Holy Spirit. It was my relationship with God that enabled me to escape being a hostage to panic attacks. As I was enjoying my newfound freedom from panic attacks, little did I know that Father God was about to launch me in encounters with Him that *would completely* transform my life. It was a wild ride, and this ride was awesome!

OKAY, GOD, YOU HAVE MY ATTENTION

Let's do a quick timeline recap:

- 1981 to 1992 – I began to press in to learn more and more about God. I was determined to go from theories to actual verification.
- 1992 – *I experienced my first panic attack.* Was there a relationship between the first panic attack and breaking up the dungeon of demonic worship? We will answer that question as we progress along.
- 1992 to 1999 – I was held hostage by my panic attacks.
- 1999 to 2004 – I began to obtain levels of freedom.
- 2004 to present – I obtained freedom, devoting a large portion of my time to educating people about panic attacks and the truth that I had attained concerning God.

In following our timeline, I provided you with information and details covering the years from 1981 to 1992, when I spent my time seeking information about God. I then covered the period spanning 1992 to 2004, in which I provided extensive information on how I finally overcame panic attacks while continually pressing in to grow spiritually. Now it's time to give you the events beginning in 2004.

By the time we reached 2004, I began to learn more and more about God, which enabled me to ensure my freedom from panic attacks and take me to the place where the promises of God would be seen in my life.

As I look back, it was interesting how God continued to answer my prayers to obtain my desire to know Him better.

In 2004, I was contacted by a man called Rick who had a friend who suffered from severe panic attacks. Rick asked me if he could bring his friend over to meet me so I could minister to his friend and teach Rick more about panic attacks so he would also be able to effectively help his friend.

In ministering to Rick's friend to enable the gentleman to obtain his freedom, Rick and I became friends. I came to find that Rick owned a gym in Lititz, Pennsylvania, just 25 minutes from Hershey Farm Restaurant and Motel, where I worked and that I would eventually own. Rick was a man of God and strongly desired to establish an atmosphere in his gym where people could come to know more and more about God.

Through our conversations, Rick found out that, during my college days, I trained people in weightlifting at Penn State to prepare them for the sport in which they were participating. Rick asked me if I would spend some time in his gym to train people and teach them about God. There were many young people in their teens and early 20s, and most of them had not been brought up in Godly families.

Well, how could I say no? I love training people, and by this time, I loved teaching people the truth about God.

As I began to help one or two people, other weightlifters looking on liked the program that I set up for the people I was helping, and I had many ask if I would train them. I told them that I would be glad to. The asked me what rate I charged.

Being my ornery self, I told them that they had a choice. Option one: my rate would be $50 an hour. Option two: I would train them for free for

45 minutes and then they would give me 15 minutes that I would use to teach them about God.

Like most kids, money was always tight, so they were more or less forced to take option two. Actually, I was pleasantly surprised by how open many people were to learning about God. We would have a blast. I would torture them in a relentless 45-minute workout and then I would spend 15 minutes teaching them about the love of God while they did their best to attempt to recuperate from my harsh but effective training methods.

By this time, I knew that God wanted me to help people gain their freedom from panic attacks, and now I began to understand that God also wanted me to teach people everything that I had been learning about His nature.

As I continued in my persistence to know God better, He actually began to reveal things to me. Don't get me wrong, I was still in search of indisputable proof that the Word of God was true. However, I began to obtain a sense of assurance that the Word of God was true, even though, as of yet, I had not been blessed with the opportunity to "walk on water or raise the dead." I say that somewhat jokingly, but as you "press in" and begin to really believe the goodness and integrity of God and you come to receive the revelation of what Jesus did for us, your belief in God and your confidence in His goodness just seems to continue to grow. At least, that's the way it was for me.

In listening to the teachings and testimonies of other men and women of God, they would often refer to their ability to actually hear from Him. This was a little heavy for me, but at that point, I refused to rule anything out.

The Word of God says that when we receive Jesus, our spirit is made alive to God. Then we have the ability to be filled with the Holy Spirit. If I'm truly filled with the Holy Spirit, then it would stand to reason that I should be able to receive direction from the Spirit of God that resides inside of me, communicating with my spirit.

I soon began to receive the revelation that this is exactly how it works. I didn't hear God with my physical ears, but I did begin to obtain the ability to hear with my spiritual "ears." As I began to be led by the Spirit of God, I became aware that my conscience was positioning me to hear from God. God leads us by his spirit, and within us, we get a type of "knowing" of God.

As awesome as this is, I still had to learn how to differentiate between what I believed to be the voice of God versus just my own thoughts. In *Psalms 46:10* (NKJV), the Word of God says, *"Be still, and know that I am God."* That sounds awesome, but by this time, we know that "being still" is not necessarily my biggest strength. Regardless, I chose to be very intentional about listening to the leading of the Lord—a leading that would come from the spirit of the Lord into my spirit and then begin to illuminate my mind.

God kept putting me in a position where I obtained more and more verification that He was the one true God and that His word was the truth.

NOT A MINUTE TO WASTE

One day, I had the opportunity to minister to a kid who seemed a little lost. He was only 19 years old, and he came from a broken home. By this time, I began to be able to tangibly perceive God guiding me in ministering to people. I put this kid through a workout, and the 15-minute mandatory God talk went for about two hours. He took everything in, but he didn't seem to say a lot. I knew he was receiving what I was saying, but I couldn't understand why he was so quiet.

Well, the next day, the kid showed up at the gym. He brought along a book with him: his diary. He asked if he could talk to me. We sat down in the little room that was designated for me to minister to people, and he told me that he wanted me to read his diary. Five days prior to meeting this kid, he'd written in his diary that he was tired of living because nobody seemed to care about him. He didn't have anyone in his life that he was able to go to, if nothing else, just to talk to about life. He wanted to believe in God, but there was so much he did not understand.

He'd made a journal entry where he'd told God that, if somebody didn't come along within a week to help him, he was most likely going to take his life.

Wow, we made it by two days. The kid told me that for the first time in his life, he had begun to experience hope and felt the truth that there was a purpose for his life. He was also convinced that God had answered his prayer to send someone to help him.

I didn't know which one of us received the most from what God was able to orchestrate to enable me to minister to this young man. However, what I do know is that, for me, the encounter changed my life. I told God that this was what I wanted to commit my life to—to helping people like this.

A couple of things really became evident for me:

- The love that God has for us must be so much more than most of us realize.
- We do have opposition, which is the demonic realm. The demonic realm works by attacking a person's thoughts and emotions. The demonic realm will continue to drive a person to make incorrect decisions in efforts to cause death, loss, and destruction.
- You can be led by the Spirit of God. You can be led on a day-to-day basis to walk out the will of God.
- God will orchestrate opportunities to put us in the right place at the right time. However, God also gives us free will. We don't *have* to do stuff—we *get* to do stuff.
- Our ability to walk out the will of God will be determined by our commitment to prioritizing our time and attention. If we truly put God first, He will make sure that we are positioned to be where we need to be.
- God refers to Himself as our Father, and He refers to those of us who have received Jesus as His sons and daughters. The Word of God says, *"Those who are led by the Spirit of God, those are the sons and daughters of God."*

I began to gain the revelation that, through all these years, God was positioning me so that I could receive the answers that I was seeking.

In the years before my first panic attack, I intentionally sought God. During my years of battling with panic attacks, I was positioned to learn how to intentionally trust and rely on God as my Father. God did not cause the years of panic attacks, but He did teach me through experience because I chose to believe in His promises.

You know, it would do us all a lot of good if we could simply slow down and look at things through God's eyes.

1. God made mankind because He chose us to be the object of His love. God gave us free will. For God to truly encounter love from His sons and daughters, it has to be because *we choose* to love God. If we were forced to love God, that would not be love.

2. God made us responsible. In *Romans 5:17* (AMP), the Word of God says that we are called to rule and reign through our relationship with Jesus. We don't rule and reign through selfish motives; we rule and reign by serving—just as Jesus did.

3. A lot of things that happened on the Earth are not the will of God. God gave us the power and authority to deal with the demonic realm. God chooses to accomplish His will through our lives. We have to set our priorities to walk out what God has commissioned us to accomplish.

4. God ministers His love through His sons and daughters. God's effectiveness is seen through our obedience.

   Don't get me wrong, God is sovereign and can do whatever He chooses to do. However, within the scope of His sovereignty, God chose to minister through His sons and daughters. Around 2004, one of the biggest things that I began to learn what was an amazing responsibility we carried as God's kids.

Well, by this time, Rick was thrilled with the progress that we were making in the gym, and he announced that we would be starting a Bible study every Monday night and that I would be teaching it. I guess I would've appreciated knowing that before the announcement, but the way God was moving in my life, I was up for just about anything. And for anyone who knows Rick, if something gets in his head, he's not going to stop until it gets accomplished.

Monday arrived, and the Bible studies began.

Rick named our little get-together the "Foundry Bible Study." I don't know why "Foundry," something about iron sharpening steel. Rick was always coming up with wild ideas and names, so I learned to just go with it. Besides that, as I said, somehow I was designated to teach, so I had plenty on my plate without worrying about what we were going to name this little shindig.

VERIFICATION! ANDY'S MIRACLE

Our start was something to behold. First of all, it had to be held at Jean's house because Jean's son, Andy, was on house arrest and he wanted to attend (of course he was on house arrest; someone had to be). So, we decided to hold it in her basement.

Well, our little gang began to gather. The first turnout we had somewhere around 10 to 12 young men. I noticed four guys over in a corner laughing and pointing at each other, only to find out that, years prior, they'd all done drugs together once.

I loved it—people on house arrest, former drug users/dealers—now all we needed were some Pharisees and scribes to show up. Thank God they didn't! We didn't have hymnals, we didn't have bulletins, we didn't have pews, and people were certainly not dressed in suits and ties. But we did have a group of guys who were hungry for God, and God showed up.

The power of God hit that little basement, and everyone there received their salvation and was filled with the Holy Spirit. People were either full of joy in laughter or crying tears of joy because they had just been set free from all kinds of junk in their life.

And so, you have it: the birth of the Foundry Bible study. Being led by the Spirit of God, I knew that the group was not supposed to be large, where people would get lost in the crowd, but it was supposed to be small enough to remain very effective at teaching and training young people to eventually become spiritual warriors.

And so, it was. We would meet every Monday—guys only. Because we had girlfriends and moms who wanted to attend, we started a Wednesday night Foundry Bible study that would be co-ed. Eventually, we picked a Friday night as well because a lot of the kids wanted someplace to go on Friday so they would not be tempted to hang out with the wrong people and get into trouble.

Looking back over the years, I can see how God positioned me to be dependent on His promises and on being led by His Spirit. I took teaching Bible studies very seriously. I would spend a lot of time in prayer and in the Word of God to be prepared for each week.

God led me to adopt certain standards:

- There was to be no canceling of any of the Bible studies unless the weather made it unsafe for people to travel.
- I was supposed to be there for each and every Bible study. Even if no one showed up, I was to have the Bible study because God wanted a place where people knew they could always find help if they needed it.
- The Bible studies were not to be allowed to become casual social gatherings. There were to be no games and no fancy refreshments. The people who were going to attend were going to come strictly for the desire to grow and learn the Word of God and grow in their relationship with God.
- People were to be taught to effectively pray for other people. People were to be prepared to minister to others.

The Bible studies were progressing along well. By this time, we were probably approaching the year 2006.

We had a good group of teens and young adults who would attend the Bible studies. We saw a lot of people receive their salvation and the infilling of the Holy Spirit. It was a committed group of individuals. When someone would fall into temptation, the group was very quick to minister to them and bring them back to a place of strength.

We were so blessed to see how God would move to bring people in who would really need help. We saw people receive deliverance from addictions and progress to develop a solid relationship with the Lord.

I would spend a lot of time teaching about faith. Up until that point, I did not see the types of miracles that Jesus experienced in His earthly ministry, but that did not keep me from challenging myself and the group as to what was possible when a person truly believed in God. Little did I know that God was positioning us to truly see His power revealed through us.

At this point, we were meeting three times a week—Monday, Wednesday, and Friday. Even though Andy had finished his period of house arrest by this time, we continued to meet on Wednesday night at Jean's house.

Andy's mother, Jean, was a wonderful woman of God. Although Jean's husband made the decision to leave the family, which left Jean to be a single mother, she did an excellent job of raising her two boys, but one of them, Andy, was quite a handful. He still wasn't finished playing around with drugs and would often take things from his mother's house to sell in order to purchase those drugs. He was only around 16 or 17 years old, but I knew that he knew better than to do what he was doing.

Andy's relationship with me became somewhat strained because it was hard for me to watch him making life tough for his mom. He was very rebellious and was not running with the right crowd. The guys in Bible study would attempt to minister to him, and even though he knew what was right, he continued to make bad choices.

It's so important for all of us to remember that we have an enemy—the demonic realm. Jesus said that the enemy comes to steal, kill, and destroy.

Well, Andy opened the door, and the enemy found his way in to cause destruction.

One day, Jean received a phone call from the local health facility located in the same town where she and her two boys lived. This was the type of phone call that every parent dreaded the thought of receiving. They told Jean that an ambulance had just brought Andy into their health facility and, if she wanted to see him while he was still alive, she had better come quickly.

It seems that some people had found Andy unconscious because he had overdosed on some of the drugs and alcohol that he had been messing around with. Once Jean reached the hospital and was given Andy's current status, she immediately reached out to our Bible study for help.

I called some of the people from the Bible study who I felt were best spiritually prepared to deal with a situation like this. There were a few guys in the group who were blessed with a "never give up" attitude towards anything that came their way. With the strained relationship that I had with Andy, I felt that it was best if I refrained from entering the facility. I stayed out of the picture but continued to pray for Andy. I assured Jean that we would be there for anything that she needed.

The doctors who assessed the situation basically let Jean know that Andy would most likely die before the end of the day. At this point, things were so bad that they didn't even choose to take him to the hospital because the doctors felt so strongly that he did not have a chance of surviving.

Well, that was just what our little group of spiritual warriors needed to hear. Within a very short time, a group from the Bible study showed up at the health facility and began to pray for Andy's life. To say the least, it made quite an impact on the doctors and the nurses who were dealing with Andy.

As soon a doctor or nurse became available, the group would meet with them concerning what had to happen for Andy to survive. The medical staff did not want to completely devastate the group with the obvious prognosis, so the staff simply told them as best as possible what would have to start happening.

Amazingly, Andy started to show signs of stabilizing. The group took each impossibility that was presented to them and called it to be corrected in the name of Jesus. The doctors and nurses were shocked that Andy continued to not only survive, but he also showed signs of growing stronger. They immediately transported Andy to the General Hospital in Lancaster, Pennsylvania, to see if anything could be done for him. Needless to say, the Bible study group followed right along.

Every time the group was able to talk to one of the doctors to find out what needed to happen next for Andy to live, they would gather as a group to call those corrections to be made in the name of Jesus.

The medical staff conceded that there was a chance that Andy would live, but it was almost certain that there would be major brain damage. Well, in a flash, Andy's EEG showed signs of life and improvement. To cut a long story short, Andy survived. Within a week, he came out of the coma and continued to be treated at the hospital.

By this time, it was about two weeks since they'd found Andy in a coma from the overdose. He was off life support, but it appeared that his body was not going to make any more improvements. At this point, he was paralyzed from the waist down, and both kidneys had stopped functioning because of the overdose. In addition, Andy had to be on a dialysis machine on a daily basis. He was not making any urine on his own.

It was at this point that Jean gave me a call and asked if I would come to the hospital to pray for Andy. The doctors informed Andy that his kidneys would never function again and that he would be on dialysis for the rest of his life. Regarding the paralysis, the neurologist gave Andy the grim prognosis that his left leg would never function again and, at best, there would be very limited use of his right leg. The reason that Jean called me was that Andy did not want to live anymore. Andy took the responsibility that it was his fault that all this had happened because he had continued to mess around with drugs and alcohol. Because Andy had messed up so bad, and that had left him in his current physical condition, he did not have a desire to live the rest of his life the way things were.

I know it may seem funny that I had not yet taken the time to minister to Andy in the hospital, but I suppose that I didn't really feel like I was in a position to effectively minister to him. I would pray for him, but I did not go to visit him.

It's a funny thing how sometimes things just rub you the wrong way. Before all this happened, I would constantly encourage Andy to stay away from drugs and alcohol. I would also plead with him not to steal things from his mother in order to have money to buy drugs.

I wasn't dealing with unforgiveness; I was just wrestling with a type of apathy concerning the whole matter. I knew that I did not want to see Andy die, but I was not as compassionate as I needed to be about his situation. I knew that I couldn't say no to Jean, so the next evening after work, I agreed to go in to pray for Andy.

Well, work was over, and I was on my way to the hospital. I would really like to be able to tell you that I was going with a good attitude, but I wasn't. It wasn't even an okay attitude; my attitude just plain stunk. I guess I just felt like I had tried so hard with this kid in the past and he just would not listen. Maybe my attitude was a little bit like, "Well, I tried to tell you."

I began to feel conviction in my spirit from the Holy Spirit about the way I was allowing myself to feel. Anyway, I reached the parking garage, got my little ticket, the little yellow gate went up, and I was off to find a parking spot. I was probably more concerned about getting a free punch in my parking ticket to save the parking fee than I was about my real purpose for coming to the hospital in the first place. As I sought out the elevator, I asked myself how God was going to use a mess like me to minister to someone.

I reached the correct floor and headed down the maze of corridors, attempting to find the correct room. Suddenly I felt the presence of God encounter me. It felt like a type of breeze met me and surrounded me. I felt light and heavy at the same time. I could tell that all the weight of anger left me, and the love of God rested upon me to replace what had been there before. I felt an ugly weight being lifted off and a type of light yet tangible anointing engulfing me.

I stopped walking for a second to try to regroup. The spirit of the Lord rose up inside of me, and in my spirit, I could hear God telling me, *"You are not here for your sake. You are here for My sake. You are not here to judge or justify; you're here to carry out My will and to be a vessel that carries and dispenses My love and the provisions of the Kingdom of God."*

Suddenly I realized that what I was hearing was the way that Jesus would talk when He ministered to people. Jesus would reveal to people He ministered to that God had anointed Him to carry out God's will. Jesus told the people that, of Himself, He could do nothing; rather, it was the Father in Him, and the Father did the works. I had to be obedient to what Jesus taught during His earthly ministry.

All the baggage that I had brought into the hospital was ripped off me, and the Word of God, which I had been studying over the last 20 years, began exploding within my spirit.

This wasn't about me; this was about the will of God. I realized that I— we—are just simply vessels that God ministers through to reveal His love. And because God chooses to minister through us, that makes us anything but "simple." We, as vessels, are the sons and daughters of Father who are led by the spirit of Father to carry out His will.

In His earthly ministry, Jesus said, *"For the person who is able to believe, all things are possible to that person who can believe."*

I can't heal people, but God can. Amazingly, God chooses to minister through His sons and daughters. For God's will to be accomplished, I need to be a yielded vessel.

When God encountered me in the hallway of the hospital, I quickly became a yielded vessel. We have to understand that we are transformed by the presence of God and by the Word of God. Our spirit is made alive when we receive Jesus, but our transformation occurs when our mind is renewed to His word in His presence.

To become a Christian is not to add something new; it is to become something new.

It wasn't about me coming to the hospital; it was about the presence of God coming to the hospital through a yielded vessel—I was that yielded vessel. How I felt about the situation was absolutely and completely irrelevant!

Well, by this time, I felt like crawling in a hole and hiding out for a while because of the way I had been behaving. Well, God would have none of that. I was being taught, and I learned my lesson very well and very fast. For over 20 years, I had anxiously pressed in to walk out the Gospel of Jesus Christ in power and authority, and by my standards, driven by impatience, I was way behind schedule.

It's hard to completely describe the transformation that occurred on the way to Andy's room, but I can explain it by telling you that I had the most amazing revelation of actually carrying the presence of the Lord. I had no concern anymore about the way I felt, nor any feelings of being inconvenienced or concerned over getting my little parking ticket punched. I just know that I entered Andy's room with a complete awareness of the presence of God and absolutely no concern about myself except to be completely in sync with the will of God so that I could watch my Father display the unlimited depth of His love.

As I walked into Andy's hospital room, I found him sitting in a wheelchair. I felt nothing but love and compassion for Andy. Anything of the past was gone, and my insensitive feelings were driven out by the amazing responsibility that I felt God wanted to minister to Andy through me.

I didn't waste any time with small talk; I knew I was on a mission. We had two kidneys that needed to be brought back to life, and we had two legs that had to regain their ability to function properly. With the encounter that I'd just had with God in the hallway as I was finding my way to Andy's room, I felt nothing but confidence in what I knew I was called to do. God's will was going to be done if I had the ability to believe. Let me tell you that, when God encounters you like He encountered me, the ability to believe is no longer a problem.

I tried to tune everything out except for what had to be done. I don't even remember talking to anybody. I took two pillows off the bed and laid them on Andy's lap. I then got on my knees and laid my head on the pillows. God was running the show; I was simply the go-between. I was just a taxi giving God a ride where he needed to go.

With my head on the pillows, I positioned myself to receive direction from the Lord. I'm sure there were noises coming from outside, but I was unaware of them. I spoke to Andy's kidneys, and in the name of Jesus, I called life back into those kidneys.

Let me interject something here. Over the years, and studying the earthly ministry of Jesus and of the disciples, I'd come to realize that, when ministering to people for healing and deliverance, they do not pray to God and ask God to heal people; instead, they speak to the problem that needs to be corrected using the name of Jesus.

Over the years, I've come to realize that most of my prayer time is used to build a relationship with my Father God, and I use the name of Jesus to correct anything that is out of line with the will of my Father. For anything that Jesus purchased for me on the cross, I would always speak his name to make the necessary corrections.

In the third chapter of the book of Acts, Peter and John were going into the temple. Outside of the temple, there was a disabled man seeking alms. Peter said to the man, *"What I have, I give to you. In the use of the name of Jesus, rise up and be healed."* Immediately the disabled man was brought to his feet and was completely healed. Peter and John did not pray about it; instead, they relied on the use of the name of Jesus. We are blessed to speak the name of Jesus to call about corrections that need to be made.

In Andy's case, his kidneys were dead and needed to come to life. I spoke to the kidneys in the name of Jesus, commanding them to come alive and begin to function. I'm sure there were people looking on who thought I was crazy. I don't think that I could have cared less.

I heard the Spirit of the Lord telling me to continue what I was doing. Then I heard the Spirit of the Lord tell me that Andy needed to ask his body to forgive him for all that he had done to his body. This sounded so bizarre to me that I knew that it wasn't something that I had come up with. I told Andy what to do, and he was very quick to do it.

I ministered to his kidneys for about 15 to 20 minutes before concentrating on his legs. The left leg had absolutely no movement, while, on his right, he only had the ability to move his big toe.

I started speaking over his right leg in the name of Jesus and called it to be healed, to be made whole, and to begin to function properly. It wasn't more than five or 10 minutes until all the toes began to move, and then he began to move his foot as his ankle gained mobility. After about 20 minutes, the power of God had his right leg functioning from the knee down. I was operating at such an amazing level of faith that the progress that we were making didn't even faze me.

I then started to speak to the left leg, and we began to get movement in the toes. I told Andy that his kidneys would begin to function properly and that, within two weeks, he would be out of the wheelchair and would be walking with the use of a cane or walker until his legs strengthened.

As I was listening to the Lord, I instructed Andy to do nothing but speak what needed to be corrected in the name of Jesus. I told him to spend time with God in repentance for the things that he'd done wrong and to establish a close relationship with God. I told him to refrain from speaking anything negative and not be moved by what he saw, but rather, only by what he believed.

It was time for me to leave, so I headed out of Andy's room. I don't even remember walking; I think I was kind of floating down the hallways. I'd asked for an encounter with God, and I'd gotten an encounter with God. I asked to see the miraculous, and then God had shown me the miraculous.

When I got home, somehow I was able to sleep. I just remember continually thanking God for letting me be a part of what happened that night.

The next day, as always, Jean went in to see her son, Andy. His nurse came running up to Jean, waving around a bag that contained urine—Andy's urine. For the first time since he'd arrived at the hospital, Andy's kidneys functioned. Everyone was freaking out! I got a call that morning. I attempted to play it cool, but I was freaking out, too.

It had only been eight or nine hours since God had ministered to Andy, and already his kidneys had begun to function. Well, to fast-forward, Andy never went back on dialysis again, and within two and half weeks, he was out of the wheelchair, walking on his own. He was released from the hospital. A few weeks later, he went back to visit his doctors—the urologist and the neurologist. Andy asked if they had any explanations; they had none. Both doctors admitted that it had to be an act of God that not only was Andy alive, but that his kidneys and legs were also functioning properly.

Well, God was faithful. I wanted to see a move of God and display of the power of God that could not be disputed, and I definitely received it.

So many people ask me how I know that what I believe is real, how I know that the God I believe in is the only true God, and how I know that the Word of God is true and Jesus is who the Word of God says He is. For the record, I never debate with people; I just give them the evidence.

I can't tell you how many people have received their salvation and received Jesus as Lord and God as their Father through this story, but it has provided me with evidence that can't be disputed. I know the enemy dreaded the day when I personally saw the display of the power and love of God and actually was the vessel that God used.

Well, we started this wild ride. Let's keep it going.

WHERE DO WE GO FROM HERE?

AN ANOINTING

Journey 1 *I was a victim of panic attacks*

Through God's help, I defeated my panic attacks and found freedom. I refused to be a victim and was committed to obtaining my freedom from that terrible beast. Panic attacks had found an open door into my life. Well, I went on the offensive to attack those panic attacks in my determination to obtain my deliverance.

I want you to be free from panic attacks, anxiety disorder, stress, addictions, and anything else that is attempting to rob the quality of your life. Use this book as a guide to obtaining your freedom by applying the principles taught here to be able to live in peace, joy, and contentment.

Journey 2 *I was a victim of spiritual confusion*

Maybe this is not a big deal to some people, but I'm not some people; I don't take things lightly.

I was determined to bring an end to my confusion about God. I attacked my confusion with the same gusto and determination as I did with my panic attacks. I was relentless in my determination to obtain the truth. I diligently sought God after 1979 and was determined to get some answers.

Through God's mercy and goodness, my spiritual confusion was beginning to be brought to an end.

Over the years, I developed a Father/son relationship with God. I had received Jesus as my Savior, and I knew I was born again. I pressed in to receive the blessing of being filled with the Holy Spirit. However, when God my Father chose to minister through me to accomplish what could undeniably not be accomplished through my own human strength and effort, questions and confusion began to lose their grip and no longer had the ability to haunt me. The way my Father used me to minister to Andy and bring about his healing completely changed my life. I say this with all humility, but what I truly experienced was the opportunity to partner with my Father to enable the desire of my Father to be accomplished.

It says in the Scriptures that God likes us to refer to Him as "ABBA"—Father. Translated, this actually means Dad or Daddy.

Over the years, I've really come to know my Dad, my Father God. I know Him through the Scriptures, I know Him by studying the earthly ministry of Jesus, and I know Him the way He intimately ministers through me in the person of the Holy Spirit. That's why I have such a problem when people talk trash about my Dad. Some people talk bad about Dad because they never had the opportunity to be taught correctly. Some people talk bad about Father because they are confused, because they are deceived, and because they just repeat what they have been told. Some people blame my Heavenly Father because they live in self-pity and they refuse to take responsibility for the mistakes that they are actually responsible for.

We started this spiritual journey, so let's keep going. I've shared with you what confusion I initially had, I've shared with you things that I have learned, I've shared with you the demonic attack on my life, and I've shared with you how I personally experienced the power of God released through me to accomplish His will.

Travel with me now as we continue and eventually conclude the spiritual journey. I have some things to share with you that could change your life. I've things to share with you that have the ability to bring about freedom from anything that you are being held hostage to. If you are interested, I have things to share with you that will teach you how to position yourself to obtain the blessing of a Father relationship with the God of the universe. The last leg of this journey is awesome, and you are going to love where it takes us.

Father God began our Bible studies in 2004, and they continue to this day. It was around 2005 that Andy received his healing and deliverance.

We started out having Bible study on Monday. Then we added Wednesday, and eventually, we picked up Friday. Father then positioned me to teach a Bible study on Thursday night in Perry County, Pennsylvania. This trip was one and a half hours each way. There was a group of hungry people up there who asked to be ministered to.

Eventually, along with the Bible studies, at the leading of the Lord, we started Sunday morning church service in Lancaster County. So, Father led me to teach a Bible study every Monday, Wednesday, Thursday, and Friday and church on Sunday morning. Amazingly, I did all this while I was also responsible for overseeing Hershey Farm Restaurant, Motel, and Gift Shop. Not exactly a nine to five position.

Looking back, I see what Father had positioned me to do. He was positioning me to do the impossible. What Father requested of me was absolutely impossible through my own human strength and my own human effort.

I was not to miss any Bible studies. I had one day off from work— Monday—and that day was to be devoted to spending time with God's Word and in the presence of the Holy Spirit to prepare for the upcoming Bible studies and church service.

I was very happy to accept the responsibility that my Father offered me, mostly because I knew that it would have to be accomplished through divine intervention, and that was the only way that I wanted to live.

If I could just interject something here. From 2004 until the present time of 2019, supernaturally, Father enabled me to attend each and every Bible study except one, which I was able to effectively accomplish over the phone. What my Father did was to continue to show me that impossibilities are made possible through our relationship with Him.

Please understand. I'm not saying this out of any self-pity or desire to exalt myself. I asked my Father to reveal Himself to me, and He honored the request. Each Monday, Father God would enable me to write a Bible study that could be used as a handout for people to read who could not attend a Bible study. Each was about eight pages long. It was an awesome tool to send people in prison, those who had moved away, and those on mission trips. It enabled me to consistently be in His presence and learn to be led by the Holy Spirit.

I don't mean this with the least bit of arrogance, but I find myself to be one of the most content people I know. I absolutely love the job I do at Hershey Farm, and I absolutely love ministering to people. I love waking up in the morning and I love going to sleep at night. All my needs are met.

With everything that I learned over the last 15 years, with all my notes, Bible studies, and journal entries, God has now given me the motivation to begin writing more books. I still teach three Bible studies a week and minister at church Sunday morning, but I sense that God wants me to put more focus on writing.

I felt it was important to include that information about the last 15 years so it will help you to be better positioned to receive some of the scriptural information that I will be sharing. As we continue along the journey, I'm going to reveal how Father God taught me to effectively walk out the ministry call, which not only applies to my life, but also yours. Let's begin by looking at the ministry that God commits to us.

Bear in mind that my questions up to this point were:

- If God is God, why isn't He a huge part of our everyday lives?
- If God is a loving God, why do people teach that He uses sickness, pain, and suffering to teach us?
- If God is God, why are there so many religions? Why are there so many denominations?
- If God is God, why do people say that He is in control when so many terrible things happen in the world?
- If God is God, why don't we see miracles today like the ones we saw through the hands of people who follow Jesus?

Over the years, I had my questions answered, and through this journey, I want *any* spiritual confusion in your life to be done away with.

After Andy received his healing, momentum was on my side. It was time to get some of the tough questions answered. Confusion needed to be done away with. As I ministered, one of the most reoccurring questions that people brought up about God would be, "If God is in control, why does He let so many terrible things happen? Why did He allow this person to die when everyone saw them as a good person who never hurt anyone? Why didn't He step in and save that person—why did He not step in and heal them?

My question is: is God really in control? Now, before you look for a cliff to throw me off or begin to search for small rocks to stone me with, let's look at some crucial truths.

1. God made the Earth, and God gave the responsibility of the Earth to humankind.
2. Humankind messed things up, and the devil took control.
3. God sent Jesus to reconcile us back to Himself and to undo the works of the enemy.
4. Jesus defeated the enemy, but He did not destroy the enemy. The enemy would be made ineffective by the power of the Holy Spirit ministering through God's sons and daughters.

5. The enemy works through deception. Could it be that the enemy causes enough deception among the sons and daughters of Father to where they don't realize the responsibility that they have?

I know the *question of God being in control* is a tough subject, but if we're going to successfully chip away at confusing spiritual issues, it's going to be the tough subjects that we're going to have to face.

My Father is good. My Father is really, really good. My Father sent His Son Jesus to die for me, to die for you.

After everything God did, so many people still do not believe in Him. People curse His name, people take His name in vain. People disrespect him, people dishonor Him. My Father is so powerful that with a simple snap of his finger, He could instantly wipe those people off the face of the Earth. But He doesn't. Why not? Because He loves us, even the ones *who do not know him* and even those who curse His name.

Well, I know Him. I know my Father God. I know His nature. Jesus revealed His nature to me in His earthly ministry.

My Father trusted me with the responsibility to reconcile the lost to Him by walking out a lifestyle of power and authority that Jesus died to enable me to receive.

Jesus made the amazing statement, *"If you have seen Me, then you have seen the Father."* Now, it's up to us to step up to the plate and get our job done. What is it going to take for us to be able to make the statement, "If you have seen me, you have correctly seen Jesus."

You see, if we correctly reveal Jesus and the earthly ministry of Jesus correctly reveals the Father, then a disciplined life of obedience to Jesus effectively drives out deception and paves the way for the *"lost"* to be reconciled back to Father.

We have to get a few things clear. You have opposition, and we were born into a war. The kingdom of darkness will always oppose the kingdom of light.

The enemy works through deception. The enemy works to deceive people of their responsibility and of the power and authority that they have access to.

Why? Because when we walk out the example that Jesus set for us, we undo the works of the enemy, and we set the captives free. And even more significantly, when we walk out the Gospel in power and authority, it reveals that our Father God is the one true God. It reveals that the Gospel of Jesus Christ is the only avenue for eternal life and that the Word of God is true. And amazingly, it reveals that we have a huge responsibility, and the will of God is accomplished when we walk out that responsibility. God is always in charge, but God is only in control when we allow Him to effectively minister through us.

We have to get rid of all this false humility garbage. We have to stop being irresponsible in the assignment that our Father gave us.

In this chapter and those that follow, the Holy Spirit is going to clear up a lot of confusion that people wrestle with, because He is going to do what He does best: He is going to reveal the truth to us.

Let's start by looking at the transformation that needs to occur within our lives to walk out the ministry that God has for us.

> 2 Corinthians 5:17- 21 (NKJV): Therefore, if anyone is in Christ, he is a new creation; old things have passed away; behold, all things have become new. 18 Now all things are of God, who has reconciled us to Himself through Jesus Christ, and has given us the ministry of reconciliation, 19 that is, that God was in Christ reconciling the world to Himself, not imputing their trespasses to them, and had committed to us the word of reconciliation.
>
> (AMP) 20 So we are ambassadors for Christ, as though God were making His appeal through us; we [as Christ's representatives] pled with you on behalf of Christ to be reconciled to God.
>
> (NKJV) 21 For He made Him who knew no sin to be sin for us, that we might become the righteousness of God in Him.

- The word says that we are in Christ Jesus. We are actually engrafted into Christ Jesus. When you are engrafted into Christ Jesus, you go from being spiritually dead to becoming spiritually alive. You become a new creation.

- God was present in Christ Jesus in reconciling the world back to Himself. Through Jesus, Father restored our relationship with Him.

- In *Ephesians 2:10*, the Word says that we are God's own handiwork, re-created in Christ Jesus. Therefore, we are enabled to do the good works that God prepared beforehand so that we should walk in them.

- God spoke creation into existence. But then God reached down, and with His own hands, He took the dust of the Earth and He made man. Then God breathed His own spirit into His man. That's intimacy. That's how special we are to Father.

- God reconciled us to Himself, and then He committed to us the word of reconciliation. Can you grasp the magnitude of this responsibility? God blesses us with the privilege to preach Jesus so that we can reconcile the lost back to Father.

- We are Christ's ambassadors. The definition of an ambassador is "an accredited diplomat sent by a country as its official representative to a foreign country."

- We are personal representatives of Jesus Christ. We are given the ministry to reveal Jesus to the world to enable the world to be reconciled back to God.

Over and over, during His earthly ministry, Jesus would refer to the Kingdom of Heaven. The Kingdom of Heaven is the domain of God's rule and reign. We are responsible for being vessels for the Holy Spirit so He can carry out the will of God through our lives.

Jesus spoke to the disciples concerning their responsibility. As stated in *Acts1:8* (AMP), the Word of God explains – You shall receive power, ability, efficiency, and might—when the Holy Spirit has come upon you, and you shall be my witnesses to the very ends of the earth.

We have the amazing responsibility of being ambassadors for Heaven and to represent Heaven on Earth. To properly and effectively carry out this responsibility, we have to choose to repent.

A lot of people only understand the word repent in the context of asking to be forgiven for something; however, they are mistaken—it means so much more than that. To repent actually means to change the way you think. The word "pent" is used in the word "penthouse." A penthouse is located in the upper part of a tall building. When Jesus said repent, He was saying change the way you think. Think higher, think with a Kingdom of God perspective.

We are ambassadors of Jesus Christ. To effectively carry out, or walk out, this responsibility, we are going to have to repent, to change the way we think to accept that the Earth is no longer our home and that Earth is our assignment. Heaven is our home. In the second chapter of Ephesians, the Word says that we are seated with Christ in heavenly places. If we are going to demand that things on this Earth line up with the will of Father and His Kingdom, then we are going to have to embrace Heaven as being more significant and more real than anything on this Earth. We are called to receive from the Kingdom of God and dispense it into this hostile earthly environment that is devoid of the nature of God. We are called to be agents of change. With that assignment, we must embrace the truth that Heaven is our home and Earth is our assignment. Therefore, we are called to be ambassadors of Heaven. To that degree, renewing my mind through the Kingdom of God is how I can experience Heaven while I am on this Earth. Unfortunately, once you have exalted the world to be your truth, you have established it in your mind as being unchangeable. When I fail to spend time in Heaven, I stop being offended by the thought pattern of the world. When that happens, I become burdened with the cares of the world. Soon I am in so many activities in the world that there is no time to spend in Heaven.

We need to chip away at the question of God being in charge and in control of everything that happens. To help you understand this, I'm going to use the illustration of a franchise and a greenhouse.

HOLD THE ONIONS

At one point in my illustrious food-service career (yeah, right), I was involved in opening a Subway franchise. A franchise is the authorization of an individual or a group to provide a service or act as an agent for a company's products. I had no idea how strict the code was for operating a franchise. The parent company of the Subway came out and trained all the employees. Representatives from the parent company were actually there for the first two weeks while the Subway was getting underway. Everything and anything that happened there had to perfectly reflect the guidelines and the image of the parent company. In other words, even though I enjoyed a Big Mac, I could not deviate from the Subway menu to serve a Big Mac at our location.

The parent company was in charge, but it was not always in control. They were definitely not in control one day when I made a sneak inspection, only to find the employees playing badminton using the spatulas as rackets, tomatoes as the birdies, and the serving line as the dividing net. Anyway, suffice it to say that the parent company was always in charge, but it was only in control when the employees followed its rules and regulations. We, as a franchise, did not always correctly represent the parent company.

To use the example of a franchise as a metaphor, Heaven would be the parent company, and we, sons and daughters of God, would operate the franchise. The Word of God would be the franchise manual.

So that there is no confusion with a customer's expectations, each franchise of a specific parent company must consistently and accurately reveal the parent company. In the case of Subway, every franchise has to be identical. The crucial point is that every franchise has to perfectly reveal and represent the parent company. Therefore, a person can actually say, "If you have seen the franchise, you have seen the parent company."

Wow, does that sound familiar? It should. Jesus, during his earthly ministry, told the people that if they have seen Him, then they have truly seen the Father.

However, we have a major problem. Heaven is the parent company, and the Church of Jesus Christ is called to be the franchise. The franchise needs to perfectly reveal the parent company. The problem arises where we have all kinds of denominations. Denominations reflect inconsistencies within the franchises, which come from inconsistencies with the revelation of the Kingdom of God and the will of God. Deviations and inconsistencies arise when people no longer commit to only being led by the Holy Spirit.

Some churches have been deceived through their adoption of personal interpretations of the will of God. You have to understand that this is the work of the demonic realm. The demonic realm works to cause deception, which thus causes confusion, which, in turn, causes ineffectiveness.

In *Matthew 12:30* (NKJV), Jesus makes the statement, *"He who is not with Me is against Me, and he who does not gather with Me and for My side, causes people to scatter."*

Jesus spent the majority of His time preaching in reference to the Kingdom of God. Jesus did this so that we could understand the nature and the will of God by understanding the nature of His Kingdom.

Then Jesus spent His time ministering healing and deliverance to the people. Jesus did many miracles. I like to refer to them as "corrections." Jesus would minister corrections to anything that was out of line with the will of God, out of line with the conditions of the Kingdom of God.

In *Luke 9:1 – 2* (NKJV) the Scriptures tell us that Jesus sent His 12 disciples out to minister to the people. Jesus gave the disciples power and authority over all demons and to cure all diseases. Jesus sent them to preach the Kingdom of God and to heal the sick.

You need to get the full revelation of this. Jesus sent His 12 disciples out to minister to the people. Jesus did not have the disciples preach what is preached in so many churches today; rather, Jesus told the disciples to preach the revelation of the Kingdom of God and then back up what you preach. In other words, the only way that the disciples could heal the sick and drive out demons was if it was the will of God and it lined up with the conditions of the Kingdom of God.

Then, in *Luke 10* (NKJV), Jesus sends out the 12 disciples along with 70 others. Jesus's instructions were, *"Whatever city you enter, and they receive you, eat such things as are set before you, and heal the sick there, and say to them that the kingdom of God has come near to you."*

Absolutely astounding! Of all the things that Jesus could have commanded them to do and to preach about, He commanded them to preach the revelation of the Kingdom of God and then display the provisions of the Kingdom of God with power and authority. Now I am going to give you a few Scripture references before we go on. Anytime I give you Scripture references, please take the time to read the Scriptures for yourself and also read enough of the Scriptures that surround anything that I reference so you will obtain the correct contents.

In *Acts 1:3*, we see a reference to the 40 days between the time that Jesus was raised from the dead and when He ascended into Heaven. During those 40 days, it says that Jesus spoke to the disciples pertaining to the things of the Kingdom of God.

As Jesus ministered on the Earth, He told the people how to pray, as is recorded in *Matthew 6:10* (NKJV): "Father, your kingdom come, your will be done, on earth as it is in heaven."

In *Matthew 16:19* (NKJV), Jesus told the disciples: *"And I will give you the keys of the kingdom of heaven, and whatsoever you bind on earth will be bound in heaven, and whatever you loose on earth will be loosed in heaven."*

Here's my question: if God was in control and everything that happened on the Earth was the will of God, why would Jesus commission people to preach about the Kingdom of God and heal the sick. If God was in control and everything that happened on the Earth was the will of God, why would Jesus refer to the keys of the Kingdom of Heaven being the ability to correctly discern what to bind and what to lose?

When Adam and Eve bowed their knees to Satan, God lost control on the Earth because He had given control of the Earth to mankind. Remember, God is always in charge. He could have destroyed the enemy at any time, but then He would have also destroyed humankind.

God is always in charge. For God to regain control, Jesus died to enable us to be born-again and filled with the Holy Spirit so that God, in the person of the Holy Spirit, can minister through his sons and daughters to have control over anything that happens on the Earth.

I use this example again with all due respect:

- The Kingdom of God is the parent company.
- Jesus is the representative of the parent company, who came to establish the franchise.
- The franchise is the Church of Jesus Christ. The franchise should perfectly reveal the parent company. The Word of God says that Jesus is the Head and we are His body. There cannot be multiple bodies, or there would have to be multiple heads. There is only one Head of the body, and that's the Lord Jesus Christ.

In *John 18:37* (AMP), when Jesus was talking to Pilate, right before His crucifixion, He made the statement: *"This is why I was born, and for this, I have come into the world, to bear witness to the Truth."*

Jesus came to reveal the nature of God. Jesus came to reveal the nature of the Kingdom of God. Jesus came to bear witness to Truth. Jesus enabled us to be born again and be filled with the Holy Spirit, who is referred to as the Spirit of Truth. All this was necessary because, after the fall of Adam and Eve in the garden, the enemy gained access to become what the Scriptures refer to as the god of this world system. The presence of the demonic realm causes deception and confusion. Deception and confusion are either going to be embraced through lies or they are going to be destroyed by truth. Jesus came to reveal the truth. How is it that the Church has allowed deception to creep back in? Doctrines and theories are the result of the attempt to create explanations for spiritual deviations and failures.

So often, what is preached in the church today about God is not what Jesus revealed about God during His earthly ministry. To preach the authentic Gospel is to do exactly what Jesus did and exactly what Jesus commanded the disciples to do; that is, to preach the Kingdom of God and display the Kingdom of God by walking in power and authority to undo the works of the enemy.

People attempt to walk out the Gospel in their own human strength and in their own human reasoning. This does not gather people to Jesus, but instead causes them to be scattered. When people are scattered, they live in confusion and ineffectiveness, which causes even more dependency on human reasoning. The end result of all the confusion is that God gets blamed for situations and events that occur on the Earth that He actually empowered us to correct in the same way that Jesus made corrections in His earthly ministry.

Father is looking for sons and daughters who will demonstrate to the world how new creations in Christ Jesus conduct themselves as they walk out the Kingdom of God in power and authority.

Well, I've not been hit by any stones yet, so let's keep going.

WALKING IN POWER AND AUTHORITY

THE GREENHOUSE EFFECT

I live in Lancaster County, Pennsylvania. We are known as the farm belt. Lancaster County is well known for its high-quality produce, particularly its homegrown tomatoes. The use of a greenhouse enables farmers to grow tomatoes much earlier than if they did not have this protected area that provides a controlled atmosphere. Beginning in December, a farmer will start tomato seeds in his greenhouse. A greenhouse lets sunlight in and enables the temperature inside the greenhouse to be kept much warmer than what is on the outside. On cloudy days and at night, the farmer will use heaters to maintain the optimum temperature.

With the use of a greenhouse, plants can live and thrive inside despite the hostile environment and conditions outside.

As we learned in the last chapter, we are, in a lot of ways, like a franchise—we are a franchise for the parent company, and the parent company is the Kingdom of God. We are born again, and we have the privilege to be filled with the Holy Spirit. The Holy Spirit is the Spirit of God. The Word says that the Kingdom of God is in the Holy Spirit. The Holy Spirit is actually the conditions and the provisions of the Kingdom of God.

Our spirit is a greenhouse for the seed of the Word of God to have the opportunity to be planted in, to yield a harvest. It is also a greenhouse for the provisions of the Kingdom of God to find a home from which the provisions will eventually be dispensed. When we yield to the Holy Spirit and are filled with the Holy Spirit, our spirit takes on the atmosphere of Heaven. The provisions of Heaven are received in our spirit, in a protected environment. Outside of our spirit is the world, and the world is a very hostile place. The world is hostile to the Kingdom of God because the world is under the influence of the demonic realm.

The Word of God is received in our spirit. The Word takes root, the Word grows, and the Word produces a harvest.

The provisions of the Kingdom of God are received in spirit form, and they find a home in our human spirit. The provisions are the promises of God. We receive these provisions spiritually, which, in turn, allows us to gain revelation knowledge. This revelation knowledge actually becomes our treasure.

> Matthew 12:33 – 37 (AMP): Either make the tree sound (healthy and good), and its fruit sound (healthy and good), or make the tree rotten (diseased and bad), and its fruit rotten (diseased and bad); for the tree is known and recognized and judged by its fruit. 34 You offspring of vipers! How can you speak good things when you are evil (wicked)? For out of the fullness (the overflow, the [a]superabundance) of the heart the mouth speaks. 35 The good man from his inner good treasure [b]flings forth good things, and the evil man out of his inner evil storehouse [c]flings forth evil things. 36 But I tell you, on the day of judgment men will have to give account for every [d]idle (inoperative, nonworking) word they speak. 37 For by your words you will be justified and acquitted, and by your words you will be condemned and sentenced.

This passage is absolutely astounding, and there is a life-changing revelation within it. In this passage, Jesus is discussing doctrine with the Pharisees. The Pharisees were deceived by the demonic realm. The Pharisees were used by the demonic realm to attempt to make Jesus ineffective. Jesus referred to the Pharisees as being of their father, the devil.

With that in mind, allow the Holy Spirit to reveal the revelation of this passage.

Jesus made the statement that a tree is known by its fruits. The reference of a tree would be a person. I could have a fruit tree in the front yard where I live, and I could call that tree an apple tree. However, if, year after year, that tree produced peaches, I would quickly draw the conclusion that I had a peach tree, not an apple tree.

The point Jesus was making to the Pharisees is that a lot of people classify themselves as being of God, but their fruits, and what their life produces, does not correspond with what they claim to be. That's why Jesus refers to them as a brood of vipers. Then Jesus goes on to give us a vital revelation:

- What is truly in your heart in abundance will eventually be what is spoken out of your mouth.
- A good man has the ability to accumulate a good treasure. That good treasure is the revelation knowledge of the Word of God. The treasure is in his heart—in his spirit—and that treasure is released through the words that he speaks.
- An evil man is compelled to accumulate evil. This man is deceived to allow himself to be fed from the world so he lives under the deception of the demonic realm. Jesus told us that the enemy comes to steal, kill, and destroy. Without even being fully aware of what is happening, this man will speak evil out of his mouth to bring about death, loss, and destruction.
- Jesus goes on to reveal to us that, on the day of judgment, we will give an account of every ineffective non-faith producing word that proceeded out of our mouths. I really believe that what Jesus is saying is that your life will end up being what you chose to speak during your lifetime.
- Then Jesus finishes up the teaching by saying that you will be justified by your words, and by your words, you will be condemned.

By meditating on this passage, so much spiritual confusion was driven out of my life. This is where I choose to tackle a tough subject.

People are always questioning why God does evil things to people or why God allows evil to happen to people, especially those they consider good people.

Let me tell you something: we were born into a war, and we have an enemy. When Adam and Eve messed up in the Garden of Eden, Satan became the god of this world. Father God was so awesome to position us to receive our freedom from the demonic realm and from eternal damnation that He sent Jesus to undo the works of the devil and show us how to live above the evil in this hostile environment.

It's time for people to press in to learn the truth and take responsibility for their lives by living out what Jesus provided for us.

A good person, out of his good treasure of revelation knowledge of the Kingdom of God, will fling forth good things. This person understands what Jesus did for them, and this person takes responsibility to walk it out.

An evil person, who is conformed to this world and held hostage by the demonic realm, flings forth evil things. Listen to me closely. An evil person will often *not* take on the characteristics of being evil. Jesus equated evil with wickedness—a wicked heart of unbelief. On the surface, a person can appear to be a good person, a kind person, and even a giving person. However, a person will eventually, and ultimately, be known by their fruits. The fruits that Jesus is talking about are spiritual truths, not fruits that can be produced through human effort and ability.

Bluntly, the reason that so much evil happens to people is that they do not take the time to develop a relationship with God and they do not take the time to know God through His Word. People live sloppy lives. When you are in a war, sloppiness is not an option.

Death is one of the most frequently used words in the English language. Let me give you some examples. So, you will often hear people say:

- "That will be the death of me."
- "I am just dying to go."
- "I was laughing to death."
- "Death is right around the corner."

We need the revelation that we have the option to choose our words carefully to bring about what we desire, or we can be deceived into believing that what we say is not important, and we will say whatever comes to mind even though it opens the door for the demonic realm to kill, steal, and destroy. People do not realize it, but they constantly curse themselves and other people.

Some examples:

- I just know something horrible is going to happen to the children.
- Every time we plan a trip, everyone gets sick.
- It's cold and flu time, and you know who always gets it the worst.
- People confess that they will be the first to be laid off.
- People constantly say that things drive them crazy.
- People say that, as they grow older, the mind is always the first thing to go.
- People will say that a tornado is predicted in their area and they are sure that their house will be the first to get hit.

Here, I'm not trying to be cold and insensitive; I just want people to wake up to understand that the things that they are blaming on God are actually the result of their own lack of revelation of what opens the door to the demonic realm to cause death, loss, and destruction. The Word of God has so much to say about the importance of the words that we choose to speak. It is not fair to blame God for the evil that comes as a result of the words that people carelessly proclaim.

We have an owner's manual; it is the Word of God.

You have an owner's manual for your vehicle. If your vehicle was not running correctly and you did not consult the owner's manual when the answer to what was needed was in the manual, would you blame the manufacturer?

What if a person said that they did not believe that motor oil was really necessary for their vehicle? Wouldn't you look at that person as though they were a little squirrelly? *How is it that, when people refuse to honor the Word of God or rely on the Holy Spirit and something terrible happens, they blame it on God? Many people often refuse to take any responsibility for their own irresponsible actions.*

Not only are people hurting themselves and hurting others around them by speaking over them in a way that opens access to the demonic realm, but then, by blaming God, they cause other people to become increasingly confused about the true nature of God.

While we are on the subject of cars, I have another one of my cool stories to share with you. At Hershey Farm, I have a tendency to keep a low profile. When people are hired, occasionally, I like to watch how they conduct themselves without revealing my position in the company.

ADVANCED AUTO PARTS

One day, a relatively new employee, Phil, came into work ranting and raving about his car being a piece of junk. As I listened, he spoke all forms of evil about his car. It seemed that his car was not running well, and in his words, it had finally died as he'd coasted into the parking lot at Hershey Farm. He didn't have any money, and he didn't have any idea how he was going to get himself or his car home at the end of his shift. In short, he was flinging evil out of the abundance of his heart.

When it was time for him to take his break, I asked him if he would like me to take a look at his car and get it running properly for him. He replied, "Absolutely. Thank you so much. Would you actually do that for me?" He had no idea who I was, so he just assumed that I was a maintenance man. As Phil and I walked up the parking lot to look at his car, he inquired why

I was not taking any tools along with me. I just told him that tools would not be necessary.

He just gave me a really strange look and pointed out his car. I told him that God was going to use me to fix his car—that God would fix his car through me. The initial strange look that he gave me was quickly superseded by a new level of "strangeness." He just gazed at me.

"What do you mean God is going to fix my car?" he asked. I proceeded to tell him that God was awesome, that God loved him, and that God wanted to fix his car for him. I wasn't sure if Phil was going to just start laughing because he assumed this was the set up for an ultimate joke or whether he was just going to take off running through the fields in an effort to get as far away from me as he could.

I told him to lay his hands on his car and just be in agreement with what I was going to speak over his car. He guardedly said, "All right," and we got started.

You see, I had a good treasure stored up in my heart—the revelation of the promises of God. The revelation of those promises was going to be dispensed through me to fix Phil's vehicle.

You see, I know that my Dad created the universe with His Word. He spoke the universe and everything in the Earth into existence and it is still subject to His word: the Word of God. Whether I'm speaking or providing healing to a person or an inanimate object, it makes no difference.

With Phil's hands placed on the car, I also placed my hands on the car as I spoke life into it, and I called all the parts of that car to begin to function perfectly. I spoke words of blessing over the car.

He asked me if I wasn't embarrassed about all the people that were walking by who were watching what I was doing. I asked him, "If I started kicking the tires and calling the car a piece of junk, would that prove to be embarrassing?" Phil said no, and that it would just make sense. I told him that was the problem, that nothing of God makes sense to the world. And with that revelation, when we concluded ministering to the car, I told him to ask one of the employees to give his battery a jumpstart when he went to start it. I told him that his car would operate correctly and that he would have no problem driving home.

As we walked back into the kitchen, I told Phil to have a good day. I never knew a person's face could be so pale—I was wrong. After I walked away and stood around the corner, he proceeded to tell another employee that the crazy maintenance man had just gone out and prayed over his car. The employee proceeded to tell him that it was not the maintenance man but the owner of the business. Phil proved me wrong; his face actually had the ability to reach a new level of paleness.

Well, when I arrived at work the next day, I noticed Phil in quite an excitable state. Someone had charged his battery last night at the end of his shift. His car had started perfectly and operated flawlessly all the way home. In fact, his car had run so well that he'd decided not to even have it checked out, but rather, just to drive it to work the next day. Overnight, he'd turned into an evangelist. At work the next day, He went around telling everyone what had happened and what God had done for him.

When he saw me, he came up and said, "Dude, I mean, Mr. Ludwig. My car worked perfectly. Not only that, but there were gauges and lights on the dashboard that have not operated for a long time, but as I drove to work today, things just started to work again."

Well, I took him to the office on his break and explained what God had done for him. He received Jesus without any hesitation and became born-again and filled with the Holy Spirit.

What an awesome testimony. Let me tell you something: whenever my life begins to look logical to the world, I am positioned to lose all effectiveness. People constantly curse their cars and kick them, and no one thinks anything of it. I position myself to allow the provisions of the Kingdom of God to be released through the words that I speak, and the world becomes totally baffled and offended.

Let's tie this all together.

I am a franchise of a parent company. In other words, I am a representative on Earth—one of God's ambassadors. I am empowered by the Holy Spirit to walk out the Kingdom of God through my life on this Earth. My spirit is a greenhouse. My spirit is the same atmosphere as the Kingdom of God. I receive from the Kingdom of God, and it is held as a treasure in my spirit. Then, out of this treasure of my heart, I speak the will of God into existence.

We must constantly meditate on the Word of God and spend time in the presence of God to be able to look at life through a kingdom perspective. If I allow myself to be conformed to this world, then I have nothing to offer to it.

God is a spirit being. We are spirit beings. We are spirit beings with physical bodies. The physical body, with all its limitations, cannot be exalted above the realm of the spirit.

The Kingdom of God is spiritual. The Earth is physical. The Earth, which is physical, was created by God, who is spiritual. The enemy works very hard to deceive us into exalting the physical realm as being more real, even more superior than that which is God-given.

God, who is a spirit, spoke this physical world into existence. This physical world still stands in obedience to the Word of God.

In *Hebrews 1:3*, the Word of God says that Jesus is the brightness of the glory of God, that Jesus is the very nature of God's image, and that He upholds, maintains, guides, and propels the universe through His mighty word of power. God spoke the world into existence by His Word. The world and everything in it are obedient to the superiority of the Word of God. There are many incidents in the earthly ministry of Jesus where He would speak to something in the natural world and it would be obedient to His Word. Jesus spoke to storms, Jesus multiplied food, Jesus cursed the fig tree, Jesus turned water into wine, and Jesus even caused money to manifest itself in the mouth of a fish. After all this, Jesus then said in *John 14* that we should be empowered to do the same works as Him.

The reasons the Church is not walking out the ministry that Jesus modeled for us are that:

- We have allowed ourselves to be conformed to this world.
- We have created stronger affections for things in the world than for God.
- We constantly exalt the world over the Kingdom of God.
- We exalt the physical above the spiritual.
- We care more about what the world thinks than what God thinks.
- We have not died to ourselves to effectively live through Christ Jesus.
- We have become too civilized to walk in child-like faith.

> 1 Corinthians 2:12 – 14 (AMP): Now we have not received the spirit [that belongs to] the world, but the [Holy] Spirit Who is from God, [given to us] that we might realize and comprehend and appreciate the gifts [of divine favor and blessing so freely and lavishly] bestowed on us by God. 13 And we are setting these truths forth in words not taught by human wisdom but taught by the [Holy] Spirit, combining and interpreting spiritual truths with spiritual language [to those who possess the Holy Spirit]. 14 But the natural, nonspiritual man does not accept or welcome or admit into his heart the gifts and teachings and revelations of the Spirit of God, for they are folly (meaningless nonsense) to him; and he is incapable of knowing them [of progressively recognizing, understanding, and becoming better acquainted with them] because they are spiritually discerned and estimated and appreciated.

I want to show you a passage in the book of Corinthians that really caused my eyes to be opened.

When we reveal the Kingdom of God while we are on this Earth, people in the world will often have a difficult time with it; they will either have to be transformed to become spirit minded, or they will reject the revelation of the Kingdom of God as meaningless folly. Unfortunately, the Church has become so infected by the world, by human reasoning, and human logic that it is often the loudest voice for proclaiming walking in power and authority as meaningless folly. It's so sad to think that the Church of Jesus Christ is so polluted by the world that the body no longer has the ability to correctly and effectively reveal the Head of the body—the Lord Jesus Christ.

So, yes, I refuse to be conformed to this world. I speak the Word of God over motor vehicles that have died and watch them come to life. I speak to threatening storms and command them to be at peace, to be still. I speak the name of Jesus and command demons out, and I speak the name of Jesus and fully expect the sick to be healed. Am I effective at everything I do? Absolutely not. However, that only reveals to me that I must increase my ability to believe, because, in *Mark 9:23* (NKJV), Jesus said that all things are possible to the person who is able to believe. One thing that I know I believe is that Jesus doesn't lie.

FINGER LICKING GOOD

One day at Bible study, a young man named Mark, who was only 16 years old, came into the group all excited. He proceeded to tell the group about a miracle that had taken place on the family farm. The family raised chickens and would get in thousands of peeps at a time. Anyway, it happened that when the peeps were being unloaded and put into the chicken houses, someone actually stepped on one of those little chickens and squished it. As Mark was heading to the trash heap to dispose of the peep, he questioned why this tiny chicken should not live. Mark stopped, got on his knees, held out his hands with the little peep before God, and said, "Be healed and be made whole in the name of Jesus."

Well, right before his eyes, the squished chicken came alive, gave out a chirp, hopped out of Mark's hands, and ran to be with the rest of the flock. I believe the chirp of the peep was thanks to God and for having someone like Mark, who had a child-like faith, on the scene to make a Kingdom of God "correction."

Just between you and me, if I ever need prayer, I want to have someone like Mark around who has not been taught by the world to put limitations on the God in whom he believes.

WILL THE REAL ENEMY
PLEASE STAND UP?

I began my quest to know the truth about God somewhere around the year 1979. I had my first panic attack in 1992. Starting in 2004, God positioned me to begin to teach Bible studies. Beginning in the year 2018, God positioned me to take more time to write books.

As we began this journey, I listed five things that thoroughly confused me about the nature of God, or at least, what I was taught about God. Those five things were:

- If God is God, why isn't He a huge part of a person's everyday life?
- If God is a loving God, why do people teach that He uses sickness, pain, and suffering to teach us?
- If God is God, why are there so many religions? Why are there so many denominations?
- If God is God, why do people say that He is in control when so many terrible things happen in the world?
- If God is God, why don't we see miracles today like we saw through the hands of people who followed Jesus?

By giving you scriptural references and experiences, I believe that I have revealed how I chipped away at these points that used to cause me confusion about the nature of God. I want to use this chapter to help you understand where, ultimately, a lot of confusion comes from and how to protect yourselves from deception.

> Colossians 3:1 – 3 (AMP): If then you have been raised with Christ [to a new life, thus sharing His resurrection from the dead], aim at and seek the [rich, eternal treasures] that are above, where Christ is, seated at the right hand of God. 2 And set your minds and keep them set on what is above (the higher things), not on the things that are on the earth. 3 For [as far as this world is concerned] you have died, and your [new, real] life is hidden with Christ in God.

Jesus came to the Earth to die for us and to put us back in right standing with our Father. But along with that, He came to reveal truth. Jesus came to correctly reveal the Kingdom of God and the Father. Jesus came so that we could die to our old nature and be engrafted into His life. Jesus came to model the ministry that is possible through a person who is born again and filled with the Holy Spirit.

To be a Christian is not to add something new, but rather, to become something new. Unfortunately, much confusion has been allowed to enter in because people attempt to get God to adapt to them instead of them being transformed by God.

A "FAUX" HOME MAKEOVER

For a lot of people, becoming a Christian is like adding a little addition to their house. Most of their time is spent in their main dwelling place, but on special occasions, like Sunday mornings and "Christian holidays," we fling open the doors to the little addition that has been added on to our house, and we conduct ourselves as if that is where we really live, as opposed to the truth, which is that the little addition is just a place we only occasionally visit. The problem arises when a person attempts to make the addition look like it is used often, when, in truth, it isn't. With many Christians, often the atmosphere of the whole house only eludes to being

Christ-like. In other words, many "Christians" want to portray themselves as living as commanded by God. They hang up Bible verses, have a "prayer room," and go to church so others can see, but the rest of the time, they live by the standards of the world.

Inconsistencies often arise, though, because of the lack of a person's commitment to effectively reveal Jesus to the world. Instead of just owning up to the truth of not being committed, people tried to explain the inconsistencies of their lives by attaching inconsistencies to the nature of God.

People are driven by human logic and human reasoning to attempt to explain what goes on in the main house, that is, the one that the little addition is attached to. People know their lack of commitment is the problem, but they find it easier to go through the motions as opposed to dying to themselves to position themselves for the needed transformation.

I'm constantly amazed to see the priority that people put on their carnal life as opposed to investing in their spiritual eternity. In *Matthew 6:33*, Jesus told us to seek first the Kingdom of God, and then everything that we need will be added to us. Instead, people seek out and chase everything in the world and then hope that somehow they can attach God to their existing lifestyle.

The enemy works through deception. Through a lack of commitment to embrace and walk out the truth of the Kingdom of God, people allow the door to be wide open for the enemy to move in to kill, steal, and destroy. Then, when they experience death, loss, and destruction in their lives, they roll the responsibility over to being the will of God instead of the result of their lack of commitment to walk out the Kingdom of God in power and authority to undo the works of the enemy. In other words, instead of bulldozing the original house over and building a new house on the foundation of being one with Christ Jesus, they want to attempt to attach Jesus to a carnal lifestyle—a house built on the foundation of the world, on the foundation of sand.

When I initially pressed in to learn about God, I quickly understood that I had an enemy revealed to me. I also realized that there was always going to be opposition against the relationship that I desired to have with God and, likewise, the relationship that God desired to have with me. Since the strength of the enemy is to work through deception, I realized how important it was to pursue an intimate relationship with God so that the effectiveness of demonic deception would always be limited.

When you really have a close relationship with another person on the Earth, it becomes more difficult for a person outside that relationship to stir up trouble between the two people with a close relationship.

PERRY COUNTY CONNECTION

The first Bible study that I had in Perry County, Pennsylvania, had the potential to be a little awkward for me. I only knew one person in the entire group. This person had attended a Bible study about five years prior on a Wednesday night in Lancaster County when he was only about 19 years old. This kid was arrogant, stubborn, and, well, just downright obnoxious. He was messing around with drugs, and his rebellion against any kind of authority was truly evident. The only reason he was at that Bible study was he was getting a ride with one of his friends who had decided to stop in to see someone who would be there that evening. They definitely weren't there for the Bible study.

I noticed this kid had a bad limp; he had a very sore ankle. Before he left, I asked him if it would be okay if I would pray for his ankle. He rolled his eyes at me and replied, "Go ahead, make it fast. We've got to get going."

With the situation that I was in, this is where walking in the love of God becomes so crucial. Within my own nature, I had a strong desire to take his foot and see if I could twist it right off his leg. In such situations, I just do my best to yield to God to allow the love of my Father to minister through me to this ornery young man. Besides that, the young man was quite big, and I was sure that I might face some repercussions from his wrath if I decided to attempt to detach one of his body parts.

Well, I sat him down, got him to put his foot on the table, and began to call his ankle healed in the name of Jesus. As soon as I was done, he got up and headed for the door. I did not even take the time to notice if he was still limping or not. When I minister to someone, I try to never react to what I see in the natural world; instead, I just press in to the Holy Spirit to allow Him to accomplish His will.

Amazingly, about four to five years later, this same kid, now a young man, showed up at a Friday night Bible study. I didn't even recognize him. He came up to me, shook my hand, and thanked me for praying for him a couple of years ago. He told me that his ankle had been healed that night. Over the last few years, God had been finally able to get his attention, and at this point, he was a very strong believer.

Well, anyway, he'd married a young lady from Perry County, and her parents and siblings lived up there. He asked me if I would come up on Thursdays to teach the group. So many times I have seen where God would orchestrate something like this, where you meet someone, and then, years later, God uses that encounter to accomplish His will. I accepted the invitation.

So, in dealing with the group that first Thursday night in Perry County, I only knew the one young man I had met years before. While teaching the group, I focused on the importance of having a relationship with God. After the Bible study, one lady questioned me about the goodness of God. She wanted to believe what I was teaching, but it was so hard for her to receive because, over the years, she had been taught how God makes people sick and causes suffering to get the attention of people.

I told this young lady that she needed to spend time in the presence of God and in His Word to get to know Him. She protested that she already felt like she knew Him. I told her that she would need to work this out for herself since I would not be coming up to teach there anymore. She asked me why, and I told her that, during the Bible study, her husband had snuck out of the house and stolen some tools from out of the back of my truck. Well, she went berserk. She told me that there was no way that her husband would ever stoop so low as to steal from someone. I asked her if she had her eyes on her husband the whole time. She said that she didn't have to because she knew the integrity of her husband and that he would never do such a thing, and then she said that I would never be able to convince her that he ever did steal or would ever steal.

I said, "There's your answer." She snapped back, "Where's my answer?"

I proceeded to tell her that the reason that I was not able to lie to her about her husband was because of the integrity of their relationship. I told her that when she commits to investing the time to develop that kind of relationship with her Heavenly Father, then the enemy will no longer be able to deceive her about His goodness.

Well, what I said about her husband stealing from me, of course, was not true; however, our interaction had quite an impact on the group. This is the same impact that I want to have on you.

We have an enemy. This enemy is going to be in opposition to our relationship with Father for two reasons.

The first reason is because of the hate that the enemy has for God and for what God loves, which is us.

The second reason is to cause us to question the goodness of God to hinder our trust in God, to hinder our ability to believe in God, and to hinder our ability to walk in faith to destroy the works of the enemy.

Matthew 12:22 – 25 (NKJV): Then one was brought to Him who was demon-possessed, blind and mute; and He healed him, so that the blind and mute man both spoke and saw. 23 And all the multitudes were amazed and said, "Could this be the Son of David?" 24 Now when the Pharisees heard it, they said, "This fellow does not cast out demons except by Beelzebub, the ruler of the demons." 25 But Jesus knew their thoughts and said to them: "Every kingdom divided against itself is brought to desolation, and every city or house divided against itself will not stand.

Pay very close attention to this passage. Jesus healed a man who was demon possessed. The effects of the demonic possession were that it caused the man to be blind and mute. The presence of Jesus, who was filled with the Holy Spirit, caused the man to be healed.

The effect of the miracle was that the multitude of people who were watching began to receive the revelation that something like this could only occur if Jesus really was the Son of God. Therefore, Jesus being filled with the Holy Spirit made Him effective at undoing the works of the enemy. The multitudes of people then opened their eyes and hearts to God.

Miracles like this challenge the demonic realm to its core. The demonic realm could not let this happen. So, the enemy attempted to put confusion into the minds of all the people who were watching as to whether the healing of the blind and mute man was of God or the devil. This is the way the demonic realm attacked this situation: by causing confusion.

The Pharisees were religious leaders. Just because someone is religious, it does not verify that they are of God. I am not religious; I am a new creation in Christ Jesus. Religion is man-made, Christianity is God-given.

In past Scriptures, Jesus told us that the Pharisees were of *their* father, the devil. The religious mind is very dangerous. Jesus told his disciples to beware of the leaven of the Pharisees and the leaven of Herod. In other words, he warned them to be very watchful not to be infected by incorrect religious or humanistic teaching.

Jesus clears up this issue by pointing out that any kingdom that is divided against itself will fail to stand. This is the objective of the demonic realm— to cause weakness by causing division and generating confusion about the true nature of God.

To help you understand His true nature, God gave you everything that you need to be equipped with to be protected from the onslaught of deception from the demonic realm.

1. In the earthly ministry of Jesus, He teaches that, if we have seen Him correctly, then we have correctly seen the Father.
2. In the earthly ministry of Jesus, He tells us that He can do nothing by Himself; rather, it is Father's presence in Jesus who does the works. Every healing and deliverance that was seen in the ministry of Jesus was a work of our Father. Not once during the earthly ministry of Jesus did God put sickness on anyone or endorse the sickness that the demonic realm inflicted.
3. We are blessed with the privilege of being filled with the Holy Spirit. In *John 16:13*, Jesus tells us that the Holy Spirit is the spirit of truth. The Holy Spirit will lead and guide you to all truth.

My relationship with God is obtained through my time spent with Him and by studying His word. I am filled with God in the person of the Holy Spirit. The Holy Spirit leads and guides me to all truth. This is why I refer to God as my Father and as my Dad. That may be very offensive to the religiously minded, but it is certainly not offensive to God.

The more intimate my relationship is with my Father, the more difficult it is for the demonic realm to be effective at causing any deception within me about the nature of my Father. Just as that young lady in Perry County stood up and began to dispute what I had fabricated about her husband, we must constantly be prepared to stand up and make declarations about the truth of the integrity of our God.

Allow me to show you two more Scriptures. These Scriptures follow right after the teaching of Jesus when He cast out the demon that caused the man to be blind and mute.

Below are three vital Scriptures to equip us for spiritual warfare:

> **Matthew 12:28 (NKJV): But if I cast out demons by the Spirit of God, surely the Kingdom of God has come upon you.**
>
> **Romans 14:17 (NKJV): The Word of God says that the Kingdom of God is righteousness, peace, and joy in the Holy Spirit.**

Through Jesus, we are put in right standing with God. When we are filled with the Holy Spirit, we are filled with the provisions of the Kingdom of God. The presence of God then becomes the power and authority to cast out demons.

> Matthew 12:29 – 30 (NKJV): Or how can one enter a strong man's house and plunder his goods, unless he first binds the strong man? And then he will plunder his house. 30 He who is not with Me is against Me, and he who does not gather with Me scatters abroad.

This passage will change your life. Look at the players:

- The strongman is us, the sons and daughters of Father.
- The house refers to our life.
- The goods refer to the provisions of the Kingdom of God.
- What binds us are demonic deception, incorrect religious teaching, and humanistic reasoning.

I am the strongman. The demonic realm works through deception in an attempt to cause me to be bound, to cause me to be made ineffective. People are bound and held hostage through incorrect thinking based on the lies of the enemy.

When Jesus was baptized and filled with the Holy Spirit, He was empowered for effectiveness. The earthly ministry of Jesus did not begin until He was filled with the Holy Spirit. Jesus died to enable us to be filled with the Holy Spirit, which empowers us for effectiveness.

Think about it for a moment—the enemy had his hands full with Jesus. Then, on the day of Pentecost, 120 people in the upper room were born again and filled with the Holy Spirit. Remember, Jesus laid down His divinity to walk with all the limitations of mankind. Don't get me wrong, Jesus is God. However, when Jesus chose to lay down his divinity to model what was possible for a person who was born again and filled and controlled by the Holy Spirit, He set the example of ministry for us to follow. Jesus enabled us to think differently from a person who is not born again and filled with the Holy Spirit. The presence of the Holy Spirit opens up new possibilities for walking in power and authority.

If you remember, several chapters ago, I talked about how Roger Bannister was able to run the mile in four minutes. Within a very short time, other people began to break the four-minute mile. Since the time that track and field results were first recorded in the late 1800s, until 1954, no athlete was able to break the four-minute mile. As soon as one person did it, it enabled other people to run the mile in under four minutes. Why? Because the example of Roger Bannister enabled other people to entertain thoughts that were previously not possible. As soon as they were able to entertain thoughts of the possibility of running a mile in under four minutes, the thoughts had a huge impact on their behavior. The ministry of Jesus enabled us to think differently. Jesus intentionally laid down His divinity so that we would be able to understand what is possible for a "mere man" who is filled with and empowered by the Holy Spirit. It is important to note that we do not remain "mere men and women" after we are filled with the Holy Spirit unless we are bound by the enemy so he can plunder our goods.

You have to understand that the battleground for a son or daughter of the Father is in the realm of the mind. The enemy continually attacks how we think. In the third chapter of Acts, Peter and John ministered to a man who was lame from birth. The man was healed and immediately was able to walk. The impact of the miracle and Peter's ministering to the people of how the miracle took place resulted in over 5,000 people receiving their salvation and being filled with the Holy Spirit.

What a nightmare for the demonic realm. First, the Holy Spirit ministered through Jesus to the 120 who were in the upper room, and by the end of the day, over 5,000 more were empowered by the Holy Spirit. The enemy had to do some quick damage control. Because the people observed the release of power through men and women in ways that they had never experienced before, it changed the way they were able to think. Therefore, they could entertain possibilities that were never possible before. It is very important for you to read through the book of Acts. In the meantime, let me give you some Scriptures to show how the demonic realm worked to attempt to put an end to what was happening.

> **Acts 4:13 – 22 (NKJV):** Now when they saw the boldness of Peter and John, and perceived that they were uneducated and untrained men, they marveled. And they realized that they had been with Jesus. 14 And seeing the man who had been healed standing with them, they could say nothing against it. 15 But when they had commanded them to go aside out of the council, they conferred among themselves, 16 saying, "What shall we do to these men? For, indeed, that a [a]notable miracle has been done through them is evident[b] to all who dwell in Jerusalem, and we cannot deny it. 17 But so that it spreads no further among the people, let us severely threaten them, that from now on they speak to no man in this name." 18 So they called them and commanded them not to speak at all nor teach in the name of Jesus. 19 But Peter and John answered and said to them, "Whether it is right in the sight of God to listen to you more than to God, you judge. 20 For we cannot but speak the things which we have seen and heard." 21 So when they had further threatened them, they let them go, finding no way of punishing them, because of the people, since they all glorified God for what had been done. 22 For the man was over forty years old on whom this miracle of healing had been performed.

In this passage, the religious leaders were being used by the demonic realm to try to stop what was happening. When Jesus was crucified, the demonic realm was deceived into thinking that they had stopped God. However, the power of God raised Jesus from the dead and Jesus took back from the enemy what had been lost in the fall of mankind in the Garden of Eden. Not only did the demonic realm fail to stop Jesus, but now the enemy was looking at over 5,000 sons and daughters of Father who had the ability to undo the works of the demonic realm just the way Jesus did.

When Jesus healed the demon-possessed man who was blind and mute, the religious leaders tried to convince the people that He was empowered by the demonic realm to drive out the demon. How preposterous! Even today, I hear people teach that healing is of the devil. Are you serious? How deceived can a person be?

Jesus cleared up this confusion. Let's look at the Scripture one more time:

> **Matthew 12:28 (NKJV): But if I cast out demons by the Spirit of God, surely the kingdom of God has come upon you.**

Jesus cleared up the confusion about casting out the demon, but He also gave us an extremely important revelation about how the demonic realm works:

> **Matthew 12: 29 (NKJV): Or how can one enter a strong man's house and plunder his goods, unless he first binds the strong man?**

Peter and John ministered to a man who was lame and begging for alms outside the temple. Peter said, *"What I have, I give to you. In the the name of Jesus, arise and walk."* The demonic realm moved in immediately and worked through the religious leaders of the day to attempt to prohibit Peter and John from ever teaching again in the name of Jesus.

- Peter was a strong man. His house would be his life, his ministry.
- The goods that Peter had access to were the provisions of the Kingdom of God. In this case, it was specifically the use of the name of Jesus.
- The demonic realm moved in to plunder the goods of Peter in an attempt to make Peter ineffective. Since Peter was filled with the Holy Spirit, the demonic realm was no longer a match for him. Hence, Peter had to be bound up and made ineffective.
- The way the demonic realm positioned itself to bind Peter was to move through the religious leaders of the day to demand that Peter no longer minister in the name of Jesus.

Now, look one more time and see how the enemy works through the religious leaders to attempt to stop the effectiveness of Peter and John:

> Act 4:16 -18 (NKJV): "What shall we do to these men? For, indeed, that a notable miracle has been done through them is evident to all who dwell in Jerusalem, and we cannot deny it. 17 But so that it spreads no further among the people, let us severely threaten them, that from now on they speak to no man in this name." 18 So they called them and commanded them not to speak at all nor teach in the name of Jesus.

The demonic realm definitely identified what was a threat to them—the use of the name of Jesus. The demonic realm attempted to bind Peter and John through the religious teachers of the day.

But what about today? It is so seldom that I come across people who are used to ministering healing and deliverance to people in the name of Jesus. The use of the name of Jesus and the access to the provisions of the Kingdom of God are the "goods" that the demonic realm attempts to plunder or steal from us once they have caused us to be bound by incorrect religious teachings.

Jesus spent a lot of time in prayer with the Father. Then Jesus would spend a lot of time speaking to demons, sicknesses, and storms to make *"corrections"* to change what was out of line with the will of God.

The bulk of the time that we spend in prayer should be to build a relationship with our Father. Then, with the confidence of who we are in Christ Jesus and as sons and daughters who are filled with the Holy Spirit, we are to go minister the will of God to the lost and the oppressed.

Jesus didn't tell us to "remember" people in our prayers; Jesus said, *"In my name, preach the Kingdom of God and display the provisions of the Kingdom of God in power and authority!"* Time spent with Father helps develop our relationship with Him and our confidence in His will and of who we are as His sons and daughters. As we gain revelation of who we are, what we have access to, and the assignment for our lives, we minister to the lost and to the oppressed in confidence and boldness. Also, we are given access to minister in the name of Jesus, and we are filled with the Holy Spirit, who leads us and guides us in truth to walk out the will of our Father.

LONG DISTANCE - THE NEXT BEST THING TO BEING THERE – JOEL'S MIRACLE

A number of years ago, I was blessed to minister to a very good friend of mine. My friend Joel attended Foundry Bible studies for a few years before moving out to Arizona with his family. However, he then received some very disturbing news—he was diagnosed with cancer when he was only in his early 20s.

I began to pray about the situation to get direction from my Father. I knew it was the will of God for Joel to be healed, but I like to hear from my Father to know what involvement He wants me to have. After all, God is my Dad, Jesus is my Lord, and I'm filled with Holy Spirit to lead and guide me to all truth, and to empower me to walk out the will of God.

The Holy Spirit moved upon me to give Joel a call. I called him and told him that God had moved upon me to minister to him to drive out the cancer. Joel's response was: "Praise God. Let's get it done. I know that this is an attack from the demonic realm." It's so awesome when you have the opportunity to minister to someone who knows the truth of the will of God.

When I minister to someone, I attempt to be led by the Holy Spirit alone. I am just a yielded vessel for Holy Spirit to minister through; therefore, I have complete confidence to minister healing because it's the presence of the Holy Spirit within me that empowers me to drive out the demonic realm and to minister the provisions of the Kingdom of God to bring about healing. The biggest thing for me—I just don't want to get in the way of what the Holy Spirit wants to accomplish.

Being led by the Holy Spirit, I told Joel to go to the bedroom and kneel next to the bed. I proceeded to speak the Word of God over Joel, and I commanded the cancer out of his body in the name of Jesus. Then the

Holy Spirit moved upon me to tell Joel to go to the sink in the bathroom. Immediately, Joel became nauseous and began to vomit. As soon as Joel told me what had happened, I told him that the cancer was gone and that he was completely healed.

The next week, Joel went to the doctor. All the tests they threw at him came back revealing that he was completely free of any cancer.

I cannot heal people; I can just offer to be the vessel through which the power of God, through the person of the Holy Spirit, can minister. Do I always hear correctly from God? Sadly, no. Does everyone who is ministered to receive their healing and deliverance? Sadly, the answer is no. Do I know that it's the will of God for everyone to be healed and delivered? Absolutely, yes. Jesus set that example for me.

I don't know why everyone does not immediately receive their healing, but I do not question the goodness or the will of God. I've seen many people receive miraculous healings and deliverance, some instantaneously and others over the course of time. Unfortunately, I have also seen people who, for whatever reason, did not receive their healing.

The integrity of the Word of God must determine what I experience, but what I fail to experience can never be allowed to challenge the integrity of the Word of God.

For me, my number one concern is that a person receives their salvation, that they receive Jesus, are engrafted into Jesus, and are filled with Holy Spirit. Even if a person does not receive their healing and their body dies, I know that being absent from the body is to be present with the Lord.

I don't spend a lot of time grieving for people I know are going to Heaven. Sure, I feel compassion for the relatives and loved ones, but the person who goes to Heaven is in a place that is so awesome that they would not come back to Earth even if they had the opportunity.

TRUTH AND TRANSFORMATION

As we finish our journey, I'm going to reveal to you how each one of my questions about the nature of God, which caused me so much confusion, were answered as I pressed in to learn the truth about my Father.

Why isn't God a huge part of a person's everyday life?

1. People allow themselves to become conformed to this World instead of being transformed by the renewing of their mind to the Word of God (*Romans 12:2*). To that degree, renewing my mind to the Kingdom of God is the degree that I can experience Heaven while I am on this Earth.

2. People do not live a life that requires a complete dependency on the Holy Spirit; therefore, people often have a tendency to walk in the flesh and not in the spirit. The key to keeping the flesh humble is engaging in activities that are impossible for the flesh to accomplish—activities that can only be done by the work of the Holy Spirit through our spirit. The Word says that those who are led by the Spirit of God are the sons and daughters of God.

3. People do not walk out the revelation that they are a new creation in Christ Jesus. In *John 1:12* (AMP), the Word says: *"But to as many as did receive and welcome Jesus, He gave the authority—the*

power, privilege, and right—to become the children of God, that is, to those who believe in and trust in His name."

4. People are taught incorrectly when Scriptures are taken out of context. For instance, almost everyone has heard the following Scripture but may not have seen it written down:

1 Corinthians 2:9 (NKJV): Eye has not seen, nor ear heard, nor has entered into the heart of man the things which God has prepared for those who love Him.

This Scripture is a favorite for people to quote during funeral services, especially when someone dies unexpectedly. Basically, what they are trying to say is that people conducting these services often say they have no answer as to why this person died because you never know the will of God; you just roll with the punches.

No, that is not taught correctly. Look at this verse when it is included in the entire passage:

1 Corinthians 2:9 – 12 (NKJV): But as it is written: "Eye has not seen, nor ear heard, Nor have entered into the heart of man The things which God has prepared for those who love Him." 10 But God has revealed them to us through His Spirit. For the Spirit searches all things, yes, the deep things of God. 11 For what man knows the things of a man except the spirit of the man which is in him? Even so no one knows the things of God except the Spirit of God. 12 Now we have received, not the spirit of the world, but the Spirit who is from God, that we might know the things that have been freely given to us by God.

When read in the proper context, the verse above takes on an entirely new meaning. Before Jesus died to enable us to be filled with the Holy Spirit, we were not in a position to receive revelation knowledge about God. However, since we are now filled with the Spirit of God Himself, we now are able to know the things which are freely given to us by God.

Incorrect religious teaching trains us to be confused about God and actually encourages us to develop a distrust for God. Moreover, exalting the natural realm over your awareness of the spirit realm will be the start of your failure.

Why do people teach that God uses sickness, pain, and suffering to teach us?

1. Sickness is not of God. There was no sickness in the Garden of Eden. There was no sickness on the Earth until the demonic realm deceived Adam and Eve into disobeying God, which thus caused a curse to come upon humankind.
2. Jesus stated that He perfectly revealed God to us. Jesus never promoted sickness, pain, or suffering as a way to teach people.
3. Jesus never refused to heal anyone. Jesus healed everyone who would receive. If God makes people sick to teach them, then Jesus would be going against the will of God.
4. Jesus died on the cross to deal with sickness as well as to deal with sin. If we are going to say that God makes people sick to teach them, then it would follow that God would also make people fall into sin to teach them. How absurd!
5. Unfortunately, so many people do not turn to God until their backs are up against the wall. When a person becomes gravely ill or when they have a friend or relative who faces a life or death illness, they finally turn to God and begin to pray and seek His help. Therefore, incorrect religious thinking draws the conclusion that it was God that put sickness on someone so they would turn to Him.

If you rely on human logic and human reasoning, this probably makes sense to you. However, God does not make people sick to force them to seek Him. God is a God of love; therefore, He desires people who seek Him out of love to have a relationship with him.

Looking at sickness as being of the devil, Jesus gave us the assignment to undo the works of the demonic realm just as He did during his earthly ministry. It is our responsibility to walk in faith to position ourselves to allow the Holy Spirit to minister through us so that the love of God will be displayed to people through their healing and deliverance.

6. In the last chapter, we read the passage in which Jesus drove out a demon to bring about healing to a man who was blind and mute. The devil stirred up the Pharisees to accuse Jesus of enlisting the help of the demonic realm to drive the demon out. The demonic realm will always work to cause deception in the area of healing because the love of God wants people to be well, whereas the evilness of the demonic realm prefers people to be sick and tormented.

Why are there so many religions? Why are there so many denominations?

1. Sons and daughters of Father have not been committed to walk out the authentic Gospel that cannot be counterfeited. Through our lack of diligence to study the Word of God and be led by Holy Spirit, believers have failed to continue to display the Gospel of Jesus Christ in power and in authority the way Jesus modeled the ministry of the authentic Gospel. Because of that, the enemy has been able to lead people astray.

    When we fail to walk out the authentic Gospel revealing the Lordship of Jesus Christ, we reduce and nullify the Gospel to where it is now, based on our human logic and human reasoning. The moment we reduced the Gospel to human reasoning and human logic, we reduced the Gospel to a mere display of our own human strength. By doing this, we opened the door to enable the demonic realm to promote and establish counterfeits to the Gospel of Jesus Christ.

    When Christians began to walk in compromise, the Gospel of Jesus Christ no longer demanded the presence and the power of God for authorization and for verification. Without the crucial "stamp of approval" of the presence of God to verify the authentic Gospel, various religions could be established that could now position themselves to be an acceptable option. When Christians made the displays of the power of God to be optional and even deemed that the displays of power were no longer for today, the door was swung wide open to invite in all forms of deception.

Denominations were never seen in the ministry of Jesus. There is only one Head of the church, and that's the Lord Jesus Christ; therefore, there is only one denomination, the Church of the Lord Jesus Christ. Denominations are established as people are deceived that they have the right to pick and choose what they believe in.

People have become deceived through their exaltation of the church above the Lordship of Jesus Christ, even though, ironically, there would absolutely be no Church if Jesus had not done what he did for us. When people inquire about a person's salvation, they don't ask if the person has received Jesus as their Lord; they ask people if they attend church.

Church attendance is not the assurance of salvation! There are so many denominations that promote that a person is not going to Heaven if they do not join their little group. What a deception! Please don't misunderstand, the gathering of believers in a church setting is absolutely biblical and is absolutely necessary. However, we can't allow personal interpretations of the will of God to hinder the leadership and desire of the Holy Spirit.

If someone approaches you from out of town and asks you where a church is that they can attend, you basically have to provide them with a type of church menu where all the different unique carnal delicacies are listed for them to pick and choose according to their individual tastes. What's worse is that, most of the time, the demonic realm is behind creating the menu.

There is an awesome quote from the founder of the Salvation Army: "I consider the chief dangers that confront the Gospel in the coming century will be religion without the Holy Spirit, Christianity without Christ, forgiveness without repentance, salvation without regeneration, politics without God, and heaven without hell."

2. Our lack of commitment to die to ourselves and live out Jesus Christ causes division. Just before Jesus was crucified, He was ministering to His disciples, and He said the following:

> John 17:20 – 23 (NKJV): "I do not pray for these alone, the disciples, but also for those who will believe in Me through their word; 21 that they all may be one, as You, Father, are in Me, and I in You; that they also may be one in Us, that the world may believe that You sent Me. 22 And the glory which You gave Me I have given them, that they may be one just as We are one: 23 I in them, and You in Me; that they may be made perfect in one, and that the world may know that You have sent Me, and have loved them as You have loved Me."

In this awesome passage, Jesus reveals two things that will enable the world to believe in God and in Jesus Christ. The two things are the unity between the believers and the Oneness we are to have in our relationship with Father and the Lord Jesus Christ. The enemy uses denominations to promote division and confusion, which hinders the world from receiving the revelation of Father and Jesus.

Also, incorrect religious teaching centers on promoting false humility, which is prideful and brags of being humble, using the claim to manipulate or control. False humility seeks attention and admiration, like the Pharisees who prayed loudly on the street corners so that people would know how "righteous" they were.

False humility is more concerned about self-promotion than on yielding to be an effective vessel for the Holy Spirit. In this passage, Jesus prays that we receive the revelation that we are made One with Him and the Father and that we will be made perfect in the revelation of that Oneness.

Then Jesus goes on to pray that we receive the revelation that God loves us just as much as He loves Jesus. This is the revelation that is needed to walk out the authentic Gospel to drive out all counterfeits. We are called to be made perfect in our union with Jesus and with Father, and we are to receive the revelation of just how much our Father loves us.

When we walk in that revelation, we realize the responsibility that we carry, and we realize the power and authority that are made available to us because of the infilling of the Holy Spirit. We are empowered to walk out the Gospel, displaying signs and wonders, displaying our access to provisions from the Kingdom of God, and displaying a relationship with our Father that is impossible to be duplicated or counterfeited.

Why do people say that God is in control when so many terrible things happen in the world?

1. God is not in control; God is in charge. God is almighty; God is all-powerful. As an act of the will of God, He gave mankind the responsibility of the activities that occur on the earth. God put Adam and Eve in control, but they messed up and gave control to the enemy. Jesus came to Earth to take back what was lost in the Garden of Eden and died to enable us to be made alive and to be able to be filled with the Holy Spirit to empower us to walk out the will of God so that the entire Earth could be filled with the glory of God.

   God is always in charge. God is in control when we are obedient to walk out the will of God in power and authority.

2. Since the fall of mankind in the Garden of Eden, Jesus was the first person who was eternally alive and who was filled with the Holy Spirit.

Luke 4:18 (NKJV): "The Spirit of the Lord is upon Me, Because He has anointed Me To preach the gospel to the poor; He has sent Me to heal the brokenhearted, To proclaim liberty to the captives And recovery of sight to the blind, To set at liberty those who are oppressed."

The spirit of the Lord was upon Jesus to make "corrections" so that the will of God could be enforced on the Earth. God is in charge, and through the ministry of Jesus, God was in control.

3. *Acts 10:38* (AMP) *says, "God anointed Jesus of Nazareth with the Holy Spirit and with power, who went about doing good and healing all who were oppressed by the devil, for God was with Him."*

   God was present in Jesus to empower Him to undo the works of the devil.

   Jesus referred to the devil as the god of this Earth. The enemy caused evil on the Earth, which was not the will of God.

   The will of God was established through the earthly ministry of Jesus, who then passed the torch to us to continue the ministry that He modeled for us.

4. God is almighty and all-powerful. God is omnipotent.

   God is in charge. The only reason God is not in control is that, as an act of His will, he gave the responsibility of the Earth to mankind. Mankind bowed the knee to Satan, and Satan became the god of this Earth. At any point, God could've just destroyed Satan, but then again, God would have destroyed mankind at the same time because humankind was under the rule of Satan.

All God would have to do to obtain complete control would be to destroy the enemy. However, because of the great love that God has for us, He sent Jesus to enable us to be made alive to Him and to be filled with His Spirit.

The desire of God is to fill His sons and daughters with the Holy Spirit, which will empower them to control and undo the work of the enemy.

In *1 Timothy 2:4* (NKJV), the Word of God says that it is the desire of God that all would be saved.

In *John 1:9* (NKJV), the Scripture says that Jesus is the true light, which gives light to every man coming into the world.

In *2 Corinthians 5:18* (NKJV), the Scripture says that Jesus reconciled us back to God and that we have been given the responsibility to reconcile the lost back to God—we are given the ministry of reconciliation.

God chooses to use His sons and daughters to maintain His control on the Earth. God chooses to use His sons and daughters to preach Jesus, to reveal the true light so that all men and women will be saved and reconciled back to God.

You must receive this revelation. We were born into a war. Our war is not with mankind; our war is with the demonic realm. The reason why there is so much confusion about our responsibility is that the demonic realm has worked through deception to make us ineffective. If the demonic realm cannot do this, then we have the ability to completely bring an end to Satan's reign.

There is a war, and the war is over us. The demonic realm wars against us because anyone who is born again and filled with the Holy Spirit is more powerful than the enemy. The enemy hates God, and the only way that the enemy can hurt God is by causing us to be in bondage and be destroyed.

Jesus made it very clear to us in *John 10:10* as to what we are up against. Jesus said that the enemy comes only to kill, steal, and destroy. Jesus said that he came so that we can have life and that we can have life in abundance.

There is such deception that there are people out there who actually teach that God empowers the enemy to steal, kill, and destroy. Absolutely not. There are people who teach that God allows the devil to steal, kill, and destroy. That makes absolutely no sense because, in *Luke 10:19*, the Word says that Jesus gives us authority to trample on serpents and scorpions and over all the power of the enemy.

The enemy will do whatever it takes to deceive us about what we are empowered to do.

Why don't we see miracles today like we saw through the hands of the people who followed Jesus?

1. Incorrect religious teaching has caused us to question the will of God. When you don't know what the will of God is, it's very hard to walk in faith. So, many times, when someone would receive their healing through the earthly ministry of Jesus, Jesus would tell that person that their faith was responsible for enabling them to receive it.

   So many times today, people are told that they did not receive their healing because it was not the will of God for them to be healed. Isn't it interesting that Jesus never once taught that in His earthly ministry?

   Jesus said in *Mark 9:23* (NKJV) that all things are possible to the person who is able to believe. The demonic realm works through incorrect religious teaching to cause people to question the will of God even though Jesus said that He perfectly revealed the Father.

   The demonic realm has to cause confusion to keep people from being able to operate in faith to be able to receive their healing. We read in the fourth chapter of Acts how the Pharisees actually attempted to prohibit the disciples from ministering in the name of Jesus. It is recorded in the book of *John 11* that Jesus raised Lazarus from the dead. Check out the following passage in the next chapter:

   > John 12:9 – 11 (NKJV): Now a great many of the Jews knew that He was there; and they came, not for Jesus' sake only, but that they might also see Lazarus, whom He had raised from the dead. 10 But the chief priests plotted to put Lazarus to death also, 11 because on account of him many of the Jews went away and believed in Jesus.

   The Jewish people did not believe in Jesus. However, because Jesus raised Lazarus from the dead, a lot of the Jewish people came to see Lazarus. Not only that, but because of this miracle, many of the Jews chose to follow Jesus. Because of this, the chief priests plotted to put Lazarus to death. The enemy will always attempt to kill your testimony.

I don't know how much clearer the Holy Spirit can make it for us. The demonic realm has to work through incorrect religious teaching to stop any act of God, that is, any act of God that is performed through a believer that is not possible through their own human strength.

The reason that we do not see an abundance of miracles today is that people who are deceived by the demonic realm teach people incorrectly.

People are taught doctrines such as that healing is not for today, that God makes people sick to teach them something, that healing is of the devil, that God gets glory in our sickness, and that God orchestrates the untimely death of someone to bring the family closer together.

Sorry, but it's all rubbish. It's all rubbish because it was never taught by Jesus during His earthly ministry.

2. It's very hard to walk in faith when you are conformed to this world. The definition of faith is given in *Hebrews 11:1* (AMP). The Word says: "*Now faith is the assurance (the confirmation, the title deed) of the things [we] hope for, being the proof of things [we] do not see and the conviction of their reality [faith perceiving as real fact what is not revealed to the senses].*"

As I taught you in previous chapters, the physical realm has to be inferior to the spiritual realm because the spiritual realm created the physical realm. People become so conformed to this world that it is impossible for them to believe beyond the obvious. Anything in the natural realm is perceived as truth, and anything in the realm of the spirit is viewed as being eerie and intangible.

It is interesting to consider what the apostle Paul said, in that whatever is seen is temporal, and whatever is not seen is eternal. In *Galatians 5:16,* the Word of God says we are to walk in the spirit and then we will not fulfill the lust of the flesh. I am well aware that the lust of the flesh often refers to inappropriate carnal desires. However, a lust of the flesh is also the demand of the flesh to have physical verification prior to accepting something as being real or as being true.

The problem is that faith demands the acceptance of the truth of the Word of God before it is revealed to the physical senses.

In other words, the world says, "If I can see it, then I will believe it."

However, faith says, "If I can believe it, then I will see it."

Blessings from the Kingdom of God must be received in your spirit and accepted and promoted by your mind. Then, your spirit and mind will enable you to walk in the spirit with such power that it will demand that the behavior of your flesh is not given options other than kingdom behavior.

3. Believers have not been correctly trained in the kingdom principle of seed, time, and harvest.

> Mark 4:26 – 29 (NKJV): And He said, "The kingdom of God is as if a man should scatter seed on the ground, 27 and should sleep by night and rise by day, and the seed should sprout and grow, he himself does not know how. 28 For the earth yields crops by itself: first the blade, then the head, after that the full grain in the head. 29 But when the grain ripens, immediately he puts in the sickle, because the harvest has come."

The seed is the Word of God. The ground is a spirit of a person. The Word of God is planted in your spirit. Notice that, after the man plants the seed, he goes about his business. He has full confidence that there will be a harvest. The harvest is a provision of the Kingdom of God that is dispensed from a person's spirit into the natural realm. Notice that, when the grain is ripened, the harvest immediately takes place. This farmer had an expectancy of the integrity of the seed that he sowed.

4. People do not have the revelation of the importance of the words that they speak.

> **Mark 11:22 – 24 (NKJV): Jesus answered and said to them, "Have faith in God. 23 For assuredly, I say to you, whoever says to this mountain, 'Be removed and be cast into the sea,' and does not doubt in his heart, but believes that those things he says will be done, he will have whatever he says. 24 Therefore I say to you, whatever things you ask when you pray, believe that you receive them, and you will have them.**

When looking at incorrect religious teachings, one can nitpick about so many little things, but they will completely overlook the most vital spiritual teachings. Jesus teaches people to have faith in God. If you have a problem in your life that is standing in your way, speak to the problem. Position yourself to keep from doubting in your heart, but walk out the revelation that, when you believe that the things you speak will come to pass, you will have whatever you say.

So many vital Scriptures discuss the importance of our words. However, you would never realize it when you listen to the way that people speak. If you are walking by faith to obtain from the realm of the Kingdom of God to be received into your spirit and dispensed through your life, it will be dispensed by the words you speak and by the declarations you make.

If you say that you truly believe something, then the words that you speak must reflect what you believe in. It doesn't take me long at all to learn what level of faith people are walking in; all I need to do is listen to the words that come out their mouths.

PREPARATION TO RECEIVE FROM GOD

We have arrived at the end of our second journey.

In our first journey, I revealed to you how I attacked my panic attacks by using the promises of God to drive them out of my life.

In our second journey, I revealed to you how I attacked the spiritual confusion that I was facing and how, through the Word of God and the guidance of the Holy Spirit, I am no longer haunted by confusion.

In this chapter, I want to make sure that you have the spiritual understanding to obtain and maintain your freedom from panic attacks. By traveling on our spiritual journey, you will be able to look back and see how the techniques that I supplied for you to obtain your freedom from panic attacks were all based on spiritual principles. I wanted to make sure that I first supplied the information to defeat panic attacks in your life to obtain your freedom. Then, in and through our spiritual journey, you would gain the revelation as to where the information was received.

As we finish our spiritual journey, I'm going to supply you with Scripture and with revelation knowledge of how to receive from God, how to receive from the Kingdom of God. We're going to learn about how to receive:

- Salvation

- The infilling of the Holy Spirit
- Deliverance from mental torment
- Physical healing
- Deliverance from demonic oppression

You are a spirit being. You have a soul. Your soul is comprised of your mind, your will, and your emotions. Your spirit and your soul are housed in a physical body.

The demonic realm attacks the realm of your soul. The demonic realm attacks the way you think and how you feel in order to cause you to make impulsive, harmful decisions that will open the door to cause death, loss, and destruction. The demonic realm does not just move in and overtake your life; the demonic realm works through deception to cause you to think opposed to the truth of the Word of God. The demonic realm also works to attempt to create an orphan spirit within you so you do not feel worthy to have the relationship with God that He desires to have with you.

Jesus didn't come to change God's mind about you; He came to change your mind about your Father. Jesus also came to change the way you view yourself. Jesus didn't come to the Earth to make bad people good; Jesus came to make natural people supernatural.

If the demonic realm can cause deception about who you are in Christ Jesus—about who you are in the eyes of God as His son or daughter—you will not walk out your effectiveness to undo the works of the enemy, and you will not have the confidence to walk in power and authority. You will also begin to question your worthiness in the eyes of God, which will hinder your ability to receive.

If you want to be effective at receiving from God and from the Kingdom of God, you must know who you are in Christ Jesus and you must know the will of God for your life. I'm going to insert some Scriptures for just that purpose.

For the Scriptures I provide, I will either be using the New King James version, or I will be using the Amplified Bible. The Amplified Bible inserts words to attempt to bring out all shades of meaning that were present in the original scriptural text. I first like to study from the King James version, and then I go to the Amplified version to gain more insight.

Let me show you a vital scriptural passage, first in the New King James version:

> 1 John 4:17 – 19 (NKJV): Love has been perfected among us in this: that we may have boldness in the day of judgment; because as He is, so are we in this world. 18 There is no fear in love; but perfect love casts out fear, because fear involves torment. But he who fears has not been made perfect in love. 19 We love Him because He first loved us.

Now we will view it from the Amplified Bible version:

> 1 John 4:17 – 19 (AMP): In this [union and communion with Him] love is brought to completion and attains perfection with us, that we may have confidence for the day of judgment [with assurance and boldness to face Him], because as He is, so are we in this world.
>
> 18 There is no fear in love [dread does not exist], but full-grown (complete, perfect) love [a]turns fear out of doors and expels every trace of terror! For fear [b]brings with it the thought of punishment, and [so] he who is afraid has not reached the full maturity of love [is not yet grown into love's complete perfection]. 19 We love Him, because He first loved us.

For us to receive from God, we need the revelation of the love that God has for us. Incorrect religious teaching uses Scriptures out of context, which generates fear, which is driven by the demonic realm to try to separate us from our relationship with our Father. We're not going to fall for the lies of the enemy anymore.

In this passage, the day that the world fears the most—the day of judgement—we, who are in Christ Jesus, approach that day with boldness and assurance. Why? Because our judgment is not a Heaven or Hell issue, our judgment will determine our heavenly reward. This Scripture goes on to say, *"As Jesus is now, that's the way we are in this world."* In *John 17:16* (NKJV), Jesus says that we are not of this world, just as He is not of this world. Remember, Heaven is our home, and Earth is our assignment.

To receive from God, you walk in faith. Fear is the opposite of faith. Fear is of the demonic realm. Faith is our confidence in our Father, whereas fear is actually confidence in the ability of the demonic realm.

Verse 19 is huge, and it is not often taught correctly. "We love God, because God first loved us." Most people read something like, "Well, because God loved us, now we are obligated to love God." No, that's ridiculous. What this means is that, when we are loved by God, we are completely transformed by His love. Being transformed by His love now positions us to love God the way God wants to be loved. We are transformed by His love, and we are transformed by His presence.

> **2 Corinthians 3:17 – 18 (AMP): Now the Lord is the Spirit, and where the Spirit of the Lord is, there is liberty (emancipation from bondage, freedom).**
>
> **18 And all of us, as with unveiled face, [because we] continued to behold [in the Word of God] as in a mirror the glory of the Lord, are constantly being transfigured into His very own image in ever increasing splendor and from one degree of glory to another; [for this comes] from the Lord [Who is] the Spirit.**

When we are filled with the Holy Spirit, we receive our freedom, our liberty. As we minister to those around us, the presence of the Spirit of God within us brings freedom to others.

When we receive from the Word of God; that is, when we are exposed to the glory of God by being in the presence of God through the person of Holy Spirit, we are constantly being changed into His very own image. Do people really believe that? Well, we believe it, and that belief is going to position us to have the confidence to receive from God.

2 Peter 1:2 – 4 (AMP) :May grace (God's favor) and peace (which is [a]perfect well-being, all necessary good, all spiritual prosperity, and freedom from fears and agitating passions and moral conflicts) be multiplied to you in [the full, personal, precise, and correct] knowledge of God and of Jesus our Lord.

3 For His divine power has bestowed upon us all things that [are requisite and suited] to life and godliness, through the [full, personal] knowledge of Him Who called us by and to His own glory and excellence (virtue).

4 By means of these He has bestowed on us His precious and exceedingly great promises, so that through them you may escape [by flight] from the moral decay (rottenness and corruption) that is in the world because of covetousness (lust and greed), and become sharers (partakers) of the divine nature.

People fail to press in to study the Word of God because they were never taught the blessing that is made available to us.

If you are struggling with panic attacks, verse two is crucial for you. We receive grace and peace through the correct knowledge of God and of Jesus our Lord. We receive spiritual prosperity and freedom from fears, thereby agitating passions and moral conflicts.

For myself, any promises in the Word of God I turn into statements of faith that I speak over myself. For example, I would make the declaration: "Through my knowledge of God and of Jesus, I am blessed with freedom from fear, agitating passions, and moral conflicts."

The word of God has the ability to deliver you from fear and from any tormenting addiction from the world, including drugs and alcohol. We have the ability to become partakers of the divine nature of God. When was the last time that anyone taught you these principals? You see, the enemy does not want us to know the truth of the Word of God because the demonic realm wants us to remain in bondage so that we will remain ineffective and not be in a position to put an end to demonic works!

Now let's look at a Scripture that is crucial to receiving freedom from panic, anxiety, or any other kind of tormenting disorder.

> 2 Corinthians 10:3 – 5 (AMP): For though we walk (live) in the flesh, we are not carrying on our warfare according to the flesh and using mere human weapons.
>
> 4 For the weapons of our warfare are not physical [weapons of flesh and blood], but they are mighty before God for the overthrow and destruction of strongholds,
>
> 5 [Inasmuch as we] refute arguments and theories and reasonings and every proud and lofty thing that sets itself up against the [true] knowledge of God; and we lead every thought and purpose away captive into the obedience of Christ (the Messiah, the Anointed One).

We are in this world, but we are not of this world. We walk in a physical body, but our warfare is not against flesh and blood, and our warfare is not done with mere human weapons. Your problem is not with people; your problem is the demonic realm that works behind the scenes to drive people to become your problem. Take authority over the demonic realm and people will stop being your problem.

Our weapons are mighty in God for the overthrow and destruction of strongholds. Strongholds are demonic patterns of thinking. Remember, the battleground for the demonic realm is in your mind.

Arguments, theories, and reasonings are driven by the demonic realm to come against the true knowledge of God. Now do you understand why there is so much confusion about God? The demonic realm works through human logic and human reasoning to cause the deception. Until I chose to fully invest in studying the Word of God to find out the truth and invest in time spent with the Holy Spirit, I was deceived about the nature and knowledge of God.

The demonic realm constantly attempts to deceive you about who you are in Christ Jesus and attempts to deceive you as to the true nature of

God. The demonic realm will work through incorrect religious teachings that are dependent on human logic and human reasoning. Human logic and human reasoning are demonically driven. The enemy works through deceived teachers who rely on wisdom that is from the world instead of the wisdom that comes from the Holy Spirit. Because of this, so many people are taught incorrectly.

We are called to refute arguments, theories, and reasonings. The definition of refute means to prove a statement or theory to be wrong or false, to prove that something is not correct. We refute demonic arguments, theories, and reasonings. We prove them to be wrong and false by exposing them to the obedience of Christ. Christ means the anointed one. A person who is anointed is empowered by the Holy Spirit.

Here's the deal. When the demonic realm works through someone who attempts to deceive me that healing is not for today, that God does not heal today, that healing is of the demonic realm, I refute those statements and prove them to be wrong by walking out Jesus Christ in power and authority. You see, I have seen the will and the nature of God be displayed in power and authority, in the same way that I or other people that I know have prayed for people and spoken the name of Jesus over people and they have received their healing.

Look at what Isaiah prophesied:

> Isaiah 53:5 (NKJV): He was wounded for our transgressions, He was bruised for our iniquities; the chastisement for our peace was upon Him, And by His stripes we are healed.

If God was only concerned about forgiving our sins, that would have been taken care of when Jesus was wounded and He was bruised. However, Jesus was lashed 39 times. Those are the stripes that are referred to in this passage. When He suffered by receiving lashes, that is when we received our physical healing. Jesus died on the cross for the forgiveness of our sins and for the healing of our body.

Sickness, disease, and torment are of the demonic realm. Look at the following passage:

> **Luke 13:10 – 17 (NKJV): Now He was teaching in one of the synagogues on the Sabbath. 11 And behold, there was a woman who had a spirit of infirmity eighteen years, and was bent over and could in no way raise herself up. 12 But when Jesus saw her, He called her to Him and said to her, "Woman, you are loosed from your infirmity." 13 And He laid His hands on her, and immediately she was made straight, and glorified God.**
>
> **14 But the ruler of the synagogue answered with indignation, because Jesus had healed on the Sabbath; and he said to the crowd, "There are six days on which men ought to work; therefore come and be healed on them, and not on the Sabbath day." 15 The Lord then answered him and said, "Hypocrite! Does not each one of you on the Sabbath loose his ox or donkey from the stall, and lead it away to water it? 16 So ought not this woman, being a daughter of Abraham, whom Satan has bound—think of it—for eighteen years, be loosed from this bond on the Sabbath?" 17 And when He said these things, all His adversaries were put to shame; and all the multitude rejoiced for all the glorious things that were done by Him.**

Let's review a few crucial points from this passage:

1. The Scriptures state that this woman had a spirit of infirmity. An Infirmity is a physical or mental weakness. The demonic realm is spiritual. In this case, the demonic realm caused a physical weakness—a disability.

   When some people are tormented with panic or anxiety disorder, they are actually dealing with a demonic spirit that is assigned to harass that person. This would also pertain to any other form of mental torment. This could include addiction like drugs and alcohol. You see, a spirit of infirmity will cause a mental weakness. It's amazing how the attacks of the demonic realm will weaken and tire the realm of the mind.

A lot of times, people will resort to excessive amounts of sleep to try to escape the torment. Unfortunately, this will not effectively deal with the problem. When a person is under demonic mental attack, they must press in to receive the truth that we learned in 2 Corinthians 10:3– 5. You must learn to take thoughts captive. You don't fight thoughts with thoughts; you fight thoughts with words. You fight thoughts by continually speaking the promises of God over your life, specifically over your mind.

2. In this case, notice that the woman had the spirit for 18 years. That's a long time.

3. Now, look carefully at how Jesus ministered healing to this woman. Jesus did not pray for her healing; Jesus spoke words that brought about her freedom. First, Jesus said, *"Woman, you are loosed from your infirmity."*

   Second, Jesus laid His hands on her, and immediately she was healed. Notice that this brought glory to God.

   Incorrect religious teaching says that we bring glory to God in our sickness. No, the only time that God is glorified is when the kingdom of light uproots the kingdom of darkness and drives out the activities of the kingdom of darkness.

   Notice one more time that Jesus spoke what He desired for the woman, and then He laid His hands on the woman.

   The reason that more people do not receive their healing is that we do not follow the ministry that Jesus modeled for us. We are taught to speak the promises of God over a person and then lay our hands on them. Unfortunately, many have reduced the ministry of healing to "remembering" people in our prayers.

4. The rulers of the synagogue became all offended because Jesus healed on the Sabbath. The incorrect religious mindset will always operate by a completely different set of priorities and procedures than those that Jesus taught in His earthly ministry. This is

because the incorrect religious mindset is influenced and driven by the demonic realm.

The rules that God instilled were to pave the way to obtain a relationship with Him. The Pharisees were great at demanding obedience to the rules when it was convenient for them, but they missed the big picture: that rules are just an avenue to bring us to a relationship with God.

5. Jesus summed it up very well by calling them hypocrites. Jesus identified the priority of the day: *"But should not this woman, being a daughter of Abraham,* **who Satan has bound for 18 years**, *be loosed from this bond on the Sabbath?"*

In this one passage, so much deception is done away with.

- Sickness is of the devil.
- God does not put sickness on people, and God does not refuse to heal people. Jesus makes it very clear: sickness is of the devil. It also becomes very apparent that God does not receive glory in our sickness—God receives glory when His power is manifested to bring about healing.
- God does not use the work of the enemy to teach and train us. God uses His Word and the infilling of the Holy Spirit. There's evil in the world. Get wrapped up in the world, and you will probably face evil.

God did not orchestrate sickness or infirmity. God does not promote it, nor does He use it as a tool to teach His children. For you Godly parents out there, do you teach your children by harming them? Do you teach your children by sending them to your ungodly neighbors to teach them?

God does not make people sick and God does not enable the devil to make people sick. If earthly parents would do what people accuse God of doing, they would be arrested for child abuse.

Incorrect teaching is the result of deception promoted by the demonic realm. The objective of the demonic realm is to bring harm to God's kids, to keep us from receiving because our receiving brings glory to God, and to keep us from walking in power and authority, by faith, because, when we do, we correctly reveal Jesus to the world!

The demonic realm promotes lies to cause us to be double minded.

James 1:2 – 8 (NKJV): My brethren, count it all joy when you fall into various trials, 3 knowing that the testing of your faith produces patience. 4 But let patience have its perfect work, that you may be perfect and complete, lacking nothing. 5 If any of you lacks wisdom, let him ask of God, who gives to all liberally and without reproach, and it will be given to him. 6 But let him ask in faith, with no doubting, for he who doubts is like a wave of the sea driven and tossed by the wind. 7 For let not that man suppose that he will receive anything from the Lord; 8 he is a double-minded man, unstable in all his ways.

COMPARE TO

James 1:2 – 8 (AMP): Consider it wholly joyful, my brethren, whenever you are enveloped in or encounter trials of any sort or fall into various temptations.

3 Be assured and understand that the trial and proving of your faith bring out endurance and steadfastness and patience. 4 But let endurance and steadfastness and patience have full play and do a thorough work, so that you may be [people] perfectly and fully developed [with no defects], lacking in nothing.

5 If any of you is deficient in wisdom, let him ask of [a]the giving God [Who gives] to everyone liberally and ungrudgingly, without reproaching or faultfinding, and it will be given him.

6 Only it must be in faith that he asks with no wavering (no hesitating, no doubting). For the one who wavers (hesitates, doubts) is like the billowing surge out at sea that is blown hither and thither and tossed by the wind.

> 7 For truly, let not such a person imagine that he will receive anything [he asks for] from the Lord,
>
> 8 [For being as he is] a man of two minds (hesitating, dubious, irresolute), [he is] unstable and unreliable and uncertain about everything [he thinks, feels, decides].

- This passage is often taught incorrectly. People teach incorrectly that we should be joyful through tests and trials because God gets glory from them. No, God gets glory as a result of us walking by faith to obtain the freedom that Jesus died to make available to us. We are to *count* it all joy because any test or trial will result in yet another victory for us to experience.

- People teach that the trying of your faith develops faith. Although Scripture does not say that, it does say that the trying of your faith positions you to exercise endurance, steadfastness, and patience.

- To obtain from the Kingdom of God is to obtain from the realm of the Spirit of God in spirit form. What we obtained from the Kingdom of God is received into our born-again spirit. Our spirit has the same atmosphere as the Kingdom of God. We receive into our spirit and we speak words of faith that have the ability to change what is seen in the physical realm.

  However, this doesn't always happen instantaneously; more often than not, the transition from the spiritual to the actual physical manifestation will take time. This is why Jesus referred to the process as seed, time, and harvest. Jesus gave us the natural example of planting a seed to obtain a harvest to describe the process to obtain physically what you first receive spiritually.

- The first time that I ever planted green bean seeds, it was a little hard to wrap my mind around how I would eventually get green beans. However, I proceeded to follow the directions to plant the seeds in good soil. I would like to say that I waited patiently, but if the truth be known, by the second day, I was gently digging around in the ground in an effort to see if anything was happening.

Well, after about a week, sure enough, the little sprouts emerged through the ground, and in about 60 days, I had a harvest of green beans.

This is huge: at any stage during the 60 days, I could have aborted the process, which would have resulted in a crop failure. A few days after planting the seeds, without seeing anything, I could've plowed the whole thing up and started over. During the days of only seeing a plant with no beans, I could have mowed the plants over and stopped the whole process. But no, I endured the 60 days. I planted the seeds, I watered the seeds, I protected the plants, I watered the plants, and eventually, I harvested the beans.

If you want to receive from the Kingdom of God, you need to understand seed, time, and harvest. In other words, you must learn how to operate with endurance, steadfastness, and patience.

Owing to a lack of revelation knowledge, people often abort the process of receiving from the Kingdom of God. People do this by speaking words that oppose what they are believing to receive.

• It amazes me how a physical seed has life within it. I grow a lot of beans, corn, and other crops, and I've had seeds that have sat on the shelves for years until I finally planted them. Amazingly, once planted in the ground, the ground erodes away at the covering of the seed, and the life process begins. This is exactly how it works with the Word of God. To you, the Word of God could just look like ordinary words in a book. However, this is not so. The Word of God is alive. The Word of God is received in spirit form into our spirit, which represents natural soil. Our spirit strips off the protective coating of the Word of God and the Word takes root in our spirit; the Word comes alive. We protect the growing crops until we speak them out our mouths to bring about a physical manifestation.

If you do not commit to enduring, to being steadfast, and to being patient, you will abort the crop before it has an opportunity to bring a harvest.

When I speak the Word of God over a person to be healed in the name of Jesus and I proceed to lay hands on that person, I know I have just planted the seed that has the ability to bring about their physical healing.

Sometimes a person is healed immediately. Most often, time will be required to bring the spiritual blessing into a physical manifestation. This is where I teach people that they must be prepared to endure, stay steadfast, and stay patient.

As the Word says, *"But let endurance, steadfastness, and patience do a thorough work, that you may be perfect, complete, and in lack of nothing."* This Scripture goes on to say that a double-minded person will receive nothing of the Lord.

- You cannot pray and make declarations of faith one way and then speak in opposition to your prayers and your declarations of faith.

One day, I overheard a lady talking about how sick her husband was. I inquired if she would like me to pray for him. Her response was, "Well, the church prayed for him, but we really don't expect him to recover."

That's being double minded. There is a crop failure just waiting to happen.

- You need to study *Mark 11:20 – 24*. Jesus teaches that the words that you speak must confirm what you believe. Jesus also teaches that if you want to receive what you prayed for, you must first believe that you have received it, and then you will see it.

People have become so conformed to this world that they exalt the natural over the spiritual.

If you want to receive from the Kingdom of God, you must follow the Word of God—you must follow the owner's manual. A person must walk in the revelation that, to receive from the Kingdom of

God, their words must reflect what they believe in and stand in faith for.

- As I said, the first time I planted beans, my expectations were a little shaky. The next time I planted beans, I didn't even take the time to check on them.

The first time that I prayed for someone to be healed and they received their healing, everything changed. Now I count it all joy when I come up against an obstacle, because I know how to receive from the Kingdom of God and I know how crucial it will be for me to endure, to be steadfast, and to be patient. I know it will be absolutely vital for me to speak in line with what I am believing for.

Unfortunately, this is not taught correctly; therefore, people have crop failures. People want to believe in healing, but they have never been taught the importance of how to stand in faith. This is why the demonic realm works so hard to promote that God either causes sickness or refuses to heal people. Under those conditions, believing in God for something is purely a shot in the dark. *This is exactly what the demonic realm wants to promote. If a person has a crop failure often enough, then the reasonable explanation is that the crop was not the will of God.*

- If I want to receive a harvest of beans, I will have to do things correctly. I will not receive a harvest if I never plant the seeds. If I allow the bean seeds to remain on the shelf in my shed, there is no chance that I will receive a harvest. If the Word of God is never taken from the Bible and planted in your heart, you will most likely fail to receive the harvest you are believing for.
- In the realm of the spirit, if I speak the name of Jesus over something to call it to be corrected that would be the same as planting the bean seeds.

If I spoke the name of Jesus over something that needs to be corrected and then I spoke words of doubt and unbelief in correlation with what I am believing for, that would be exactly like planting the seeds, although I would be physically ripping them out of the ground before they had an opportunity to take root, grow, and bring a harvest.

It is so amazing how people have become so conformed to this natural realm. By being conformed to the world, people exalt the conditions of the world—the physical realm—over the superiority of the Kingdom of God—the spiritual realm.

Remember, statistics show that 80% of an average person's thoughts are negative. That means that if they do not renew their mind to the Kingdom of God to think in line with the Kingdom of God, then it is probable that at least 80% of their words will be negative and support death, loss, and destruction. Jesus said that he came so we could have abundant life. Jesus said that the enemy comes to steal, kill, and destroy.

God doesn't bring evil on us; people bring evil on themselves by being conformed to the demonic realm.

In the natural realm, if I walked up and kicked the tires of my truck and called it a piece of junk, no one would be the least bit uncomfortable with that. Why? Because I would be engaged in an activity that confirmed the way the world thinks. If I walked up to my truck and blessed it in the name of Jesus and spoke well over my truck, people would look at me like I was an alien from another planet. Actually, they would be right. I am in this world, but I am not of this world. I refuse to speak any words that will serve as an open door for the demonic realm to move in and cause death, loss, and destruction.

People are constantly blaming God for the bad things that happen to them. All I have to do is listen to the words that they speak, and I will know what brought about the calamity in their life.

CAN YOU HEAR ME NOW?

One day, my friend was complaining that he had to go to get his cell phone fixed because it had stopped working. I told him to give it to me, and he asked why. I told him that I was going to speak life into it so that it would work correctly. He responded, "You can't do that," to which I replied, "Let's see." Well, I took the cell phone in my hands, I spoke life into it, and then I handed it back to him. He just laughed at me. I told him, "When you're done laughing, give your wife a call and tell her your cell phone is working again." I walked away and thanked God for the access that we have to the provisions of the Kingdom of God. About 15 minutes later, I returned to find that he was no longer laughing.

It would've been so much fun to be on the scene when Jesus multiplied the two loaves and five fishes that ended up feeding thousands of people. I would have loved to watch the expressions on the faces of the people.

Jesus never allowed himself to be restricted to natural limitations during His earthly ministry. If you read the passage of the multiplication of the loaves and fishes in your Bible, you will notice that the multiplication happened through the hands of the disciples. Jesus would make sure that the disciples were involved in the display of the miracles that he performed so they would eventually be able to think differently from the world, to think in line with the access that we have to the provisions of the Kingdom of God.

You know, Jesus never reprimanded anyone for walking in faith that was too extreme. Jesus did not prohibit Peter from attempting to walk on water. When people were healed in the earthly ministry of Jesus, He continually proclaimed that it was their faith that enabled them to be healed.

In the earthly ministry of Jesus, He made the statement that He perfectly revealed the Father. Why is it that the Father that Jesus revealed is not the same Father that is preached from so many church pulpits?

The book of Proverbs is the wisdom of God. Allow me to show you one of my favorite Proverbs:

> **Proverbs 4:20 – 23 (NKJV): My son, attend to my words; consent and submit to my sayings. 21 Let them not depart from your sight; keep them in the center of your heart. 22 For they are life to those who find them, healing and health to all their flesh. 23 Keep and guard your heart with all vigilance and above all that you guard, for out of it flow the springs of life.**

The Holy Spirit is telling us the importance of being in agreement with the Word of God, of submitting yourself to the Word of God.

Don't let the Word of God out of your sight. In other words, always look at the world through a kingdom perspective. Do not allow the limitations of the world to limit you. Any limitation in the world can be overcome by the provisions of the Kingdom of God.

Keep the Word in your heart. The Word of God is life for all those who find it in their heart—in their spirit man. Not only that, when you find the Word of God in your heart, it will bring about healing and health to all your flesh.

Above all, you guard, guard your heart, guard your spirit man. Be influenced by the Word of God and by the Holy Spirit, not by the world.

When you are filled with the Holy Spirit and when you submit to the Word of God, you become filled with abundant life. Then, out of your spirit will flow rivers of living water (*John 7:38*).

It is so crucial that you are aware of what you are hearing. The demonic realm constantly attempts to feed us lies and deception through secular music. The enemy hides words of death, loss, and destruction in the lyrics of so many songs. When you allow the words to enter your mind and infect your spirit man, then, eventually, those words will be spoken out of your mouth to invite the destructive works of the enemy into your life.

If what I am speaking does not line up with what I am believing I will receive from the Kingdom of God, then I will fail to receive.

People find it so easy to blame God for all the evil that occurs in the world. God is not responsible for the evil—we are. One way or another, people open the door for evil to occur. You are either going to open the door for evil or you're going to open the door to be blessed. God is not causing the evil; God has done everything possible to provide a way of escape for you.

Don't blame God for evil that occurs in your life if you do not choose to honor the instructions that we receive in His word.

We have to take responsibility for what happens in our lives. Take a look at this very crucial Scripture:

> Ephesians 6:10 – 17 (NKJV): Finally, my brethren, be strong in the Lord and in the power of His might. 11 Put on the whole armor of God, that you may be able to stand against the wiles of the devil. 12 For we do not wrestle against flesh and blood, but against principalities, against powers, against the rulers of the darkness of this age, against spiritual hosts of wickedness in the heavenly places. 13 Therefore take up the whole armor of God, that you may be able to withstand in the evil day, and having done all, to stand.
>
> 14 Stand therefore, having girded your waist with truth, having put on the breastplate of righteousness, 15 and having shod your feet with the preparation of the gospel of peace; 16 above all, taking the shield of faith with which you will be able to quench all the fiery darts of the wicked one. 17And take the helmet of salvation, and the sword of the Spirit, which is the word of God.

As the apostle Paul begins to sum up the book of Ephesians, he gives us some amazing instructions:

- Be strong in the Lord. The amplified version says that we are empowered through our union with Him. Let me tell you, you don't get any more powerful than God. He is not holding out on us. He is offering us access to everything that we need. If you choose not to be empowered with His strength, you will be forced to rely on your own strength. FYI—your own strength is not going to cut it to engage against the demonic warfare that we face.

- We are to put on the whole armor of God to stand against the attacks of the enemy. How do people say that God allows the enemy to bring harm to them when God offers His armor for protection against the enemy?

Do people know what the armor of God is? Do people know how to put on the whole armor of God? These are vital spiritual truths that need to be taught.

- Our fight is not against people, not against flesh and blood. Our fight is against the demonic realm that manifests itself in the lives of people to cause destruction in their own lives and in the lives of others. Your fight is not against people; instead, you are to engage in war against the demonic realm.
- We are to take the shield of faith to stop the fiery darts of the enemy. The fiery darts of the enemy are demonic thoughts that are positioned to lodge in your mind to affect the way you think. The demonic realm attempts to continually lodge incorrect and harmful thoughts into your mind until an evil stronghold, and evil pattern of thinking, is established.

When demonic thoughts get past our shield of faith and become embedded in our mind, verse 17 tells us we have access to the sword of the Spirit, which is the Word of God. You use the Word of God like you would a dagger to dig out any incorrect thoughts that have been able to control the way you think. The Word of God, when studied and meditated on, has the ability to locate incorrect thoughts and to uproot those thoughts by renewing your mind.

Believe me, I am in no way trying to offend you; I just want to interject truth to jar the way you think to enable you to identify any incorrect thought patterns. The way that you have been trained to think is the way you're going to perceive God. How you perceive God will determine your ability to trust God. Your ability to trust God will determine your relationship with Him. Your relationship with God will determine your ability to believe, and Jesus said that all things are possible to the person who is able to believe.

Throughout the world, so many people find themselves facing a life-and-death situation. There are people with terminal illnesses, debilitating mental torments, and addictions to things in the world that have made their lives ineffective and have totally robbed them of the quality of their lives.

Over the last 40 years, I have pressed in to the Word of God and have yielded to the Holy Spirit to obtain the truth. That truth enables me to not be moved by what I see in the natural world, but to be moved only by what I believe based on my relationship with my Father. It's time to see people healed and delivered just the way they received through the ministry of Jesus.

Can you see past the obvious? Can you look past the natural to exalt the realm of the spirit?

Do the words that you speak confirm a divine perspective or conformity to the world?

Does the world get your attention, or do you get the world's attention?

Can God love someone through your life even if you don't?

Are you too comfortable and conditioned to be a victim that you do not have the ability to emerge as a victor?

Love confirms who I am—who I am confirms that I am loved.

Opinions are not needed when truth is available.

In the next chapter, I'm going to give you instructions based on the Word of God on how to receive from God.

Someone once said that is easier for God to get us into Heaven than to get Heaven into us.

OUR JOURNEY IS NEARING ITS END

I have enjoyed revealing to you the journey that I traveled to learn to know my Father. Through dependence on the Word of God and by the guidance of the Holy Spirit, I'm continuing to learn how to be more and more effective to be able to walk out the Kingdom of God while I am on this Earth.

In this chapter, I really wanted to challenge the way you think. Jesus came to the Earth and walked out an earthly ministry to enable us to think differently than the world. When Roger Bannister broke the four-minute mile, it enabled other people to break the four-minute mile. When Jesus revealed to us how to live in this world effectively by living above the evil in this world, He enabled us to think differently so that we could believe differently so that we could behave differently.

When ministering to people for them to receive their healing or deliverance, I share the Word of God with them to make sure they are not under the influence of demonic deception. I want to make sure they are prepared to walk by faith to enable them to believe, which will enable them to receive. I believe I have provided you with information that will help you receive from the provisions of the Kingdom of God. Let's take everything that we have learned from the Word of God and press in to bring glory to God as we receive what He provided for us.

HOW TO RECEIVE FROM GOD

We receive from our Father and from the provisions of His Kingdom through prayer to our Father in the name of Jesus and declarations of faith spoken in the name of Jesus.

Our effectiveness in receiving from our Father is so much determined by the relationship that we have pressed in to establish with Him.

Over the years, I have learned that most of my prayer time spent with Father is done with the purpose of obtaining the relationship with my Father that He desires to have with me. My prayer time with Father is also to gain revelation of His will for certain situations.

There are certain things that Jesus died on the cross to obtain for me. Some of those things include my relationship with Father, and some others are for the ministry that Jesus called us to.

The things that Jesus died for that involve my relationship with Father are my salvation, forgiveness of any sin, and the privilege to be reconciled with my Father again.

Jesus gives us the authority to use his name to obtain the things that He died for and to equip us within the ministry that he has assigned me and others to do. I will use the name of Jesus to drive out sickness and disease, to undo the works of the enemy, and to drive the enemy out.

In my time of prayer with Father, I am blessed with being able to develop a relationship with Him. I will pray for His will for such things as where I should work and where I should live.

I do not pray about things that Jesus died on the cross for because I know they are the will of my Father. I know that healing is of my Father, along with things like deliverance and the provisions I need.

A lot of people pray for God to be with us. Why would people pray for Him to be with them if, as Father said in His word, He would never leave us or never forsake us?

We need the revelation that, as we minister in the name of Jesus, we bring glory to Jesus, which honors and glorifies our Father. In *John 16*, Jesus told the disciples that it would be better for them if he went to be with the Father because then it would be possible for us to be filled with the Holy Spirit.

> John 16:12 – 15 (AMP): I have still many things to say to you, but you are not able to bear them or to take them upon you or to grasp them now. 13 But when He, the Spirit of Truth (the Truth-giving Spirit) comes, He will guide you into all the Truth (the whole, full Truth). For He will not speak His own message [on His own authority]; but He will tell whatever He hears [from the Father; He will give the message that has been given to Him], and He will announce and declare to you the things that are to come [that will happen in the future]. 14 He will honor and glorify Me, because He will take of (receive, draw upon) what is Mine and will reveal (declare, disclose, transmit) it to you. 15 Everything that the Father has is Mine. That is what I meant when I said that He [the Spirit] will take the things that are Mine and will reveal (declare, disclose, transmit) it to you.

Our dependency on the Holy Spirit is huge. The Holy Spirit will enable us to receive instruction from Jesus, to lead and guide us to all truth, and to honor and glorify Jesus's as the Holy Spirit empowers us to receive what

Jesus received from the Father. With Jesus's instruction, we have the power and authority to walk out the earthly ministry that Jesus modeled for us. Let's look at a few examples of how the apostles and disciples walked out that ministry:

> **Acts 3:6 (NKJV):** Then Peter said, "Silver and gold I do not have, but what I do have I give you: In the use of the name of Jesus Christ of Nazareth, rise up and walk."
>
> **Acts 9:17 (NKJV):** And Ananias went his way and entered the house; and laying his hands on him he said, "Brother Saul, the Lord Jesus, who appeared to you on the road as you came, has sent me that you may receive your sight and be filled with the Holy Spirit."
>
> **Acts 9:33 – 43 (NKJV):** There he found a certain man named Aeneas, who had been bedridden eight years and was paralyzed. 34 And Peter said to him, "Aeneas, Jesus the Christ heals you. Arise and make your bed." Then he arose immediately. 35 So all who dwelt at Lydda and Sharon saw him and turned to the Lord. 36 At Joppa there was a certain disciple named Tabitha, which is translated Dorcas. This woman was full of good works and charitable deeds which she did.

> 37 But it happened in those days that she became sick and died. When they had washed her, they laid her in an upper room. 38 And since Lydda was near Joppa, and the disciples had heard that Peter was there, they sent two men to him, imploring him not to delay in coming to them. 39 Then Peter arose and went with them. When he had come, they brought him to the upper room. And all the widows stood by him weeping, showing the tunics and garments which Dorcas had made while she was with them. 40 But Peter put them all out, and knelt down and prayed. And turning to the body he said, "Tabitha, arise." And she opened her eyes, and when she saw Peter she sat up. 41 Then he gave her his hand and lifted her up; and when he had called the saints and widows, he presented her alive. 42 And it became known throughout all Joppa, and many believed on the Lord. 43 So it was that he stayed many days in Joppa with Simon, a tanner.

The apostles were blessed to minister in the name of Jesus. In the name of Jesus, people were healed and raised from the dead. Look at the results of the display of power and authority: it enabled many people to turn to God and to believe in God.

Incorrect religious teaching says that God is glorified in our sickness. No, God is glorified when we minister in the name of Jesus to undo the works of the enemy.

> John 15:7 – 8 (AMP): If you live in Me [abide vitally united to Me] and My words remain in you and continue to live in your hearts, ask whatever you will, and it shall be done for you. 8 When you bear (produce) much fruit, My Father is honored and glorified, and you show and prove yourselves to be true followers of Mine.

Do you live your life in vital union with Jesus? Does the Word of God remain and live in your heart? If you do, and if it does, then Jesus says that you will ask whatever you will and it will be done for you.

I'm giving you these Scriptures to reveal the will of God for your life and for the ministry that He has called you to. When you know the truth about God, it enables you to trust God, which enables you to believe Him. Jesus said that all things are possible for the person who is able to believe.

Salvation

The Word of God says that it is the will of God for all to be saved. In other words, it is through the will of the Father that all men and women are to receive their eternal salvation. When I minister salvation to someone, I never question whether or not it's God's will.

> Luke 15:1 – 7 (NKJV): Then all the tax collectors and the sinners drew near to Him to hear Him. 2 And the Pharisees and scribes complained, saying, "This Man receives sinners and eats with them." 3 So He spoke this parable to them, saying: 4 "What man of you, having a hundred sheep, if he loses one of them, does not leave the ninety-nine in the wilderness, and go after the one which is lost until he finds it? 5 And when he has found it, he lays it on his shoulders, rejoicing. 6 And when he comes home, he calls together his friends and neighbors, saying to them, 'Rejoice with me, for I have found my sheep which was lost!' 7 I say to you that likewise there will be more joy in heaven over one sinner who repents than over ninety-nine just persons who need no repentance.

This reveals the heart of those with an incorrect religious mindset versus the heart of Jesus. He always focused and still focuses on the lost.

Ministering to someone who is not yet born again and reconciled back to Father is probably my favorite assignment from Father. Why? Because I know my Father's heart, and I know the love that He has for the lost. In addition, this Scripture reveals that Heaven erupts in joy at the salvation of the lost. I mean, come on, Heaven has got to be a pretty joyful place. To think that I can be used by the Holy Spirit to bring joy to my Father and to the atmosphere of Heaven—wow, what could possibly be better than that?

> Luke 15:8 – 10 (NKJV): "Or what woman, having ten silver coins, if she loses one coin, does not light a lamp, sweep the house, and search carefully until she finds it? 9 And when she has found it, she calls her friends and neighbors together, saying, 'Rejoice with me, for I have found the piece which I lost!' 10 Likewise, I say to you, there is joy in the presence of the angels of God over one sinner who repents."

I love this passage. I don't care how many people are around me that are saved—my heart and my focus always reaches out to those who are lost. Look at what this woman did; she lit the lamp—that means to be led by

Holy Spirit—and she swept the house—that means getting the clutter out of your life.

If we're going to correctly minister to the lost, we have to be led by the Holy Spirit, and our lives have to be free of clutter to be able to see what the Holy Spirit wants to reveal to us. Don't allow your life to be like a truck that is towing numerous trailers behind it. Get rid of the junk in your life. Be streamlined, be unencumbered, and be prepared to move when the Holy Spirit reveals an assignment to you.

For a person to receive their salvation, I have them pray this prayer along with me. I always tell the person that if they have any question about what they are praying for, they should make sure that we talk about it until they understand. Here is a sample of the prayer I use for a person to receive their salvation.

God, I want you to be my Father. Forgive me for all the wrong and evil things that I've done in my life. I understand that Jesus died for me so I can be forgiven and I can be reconciled back to you Father. I receive Jesus as my Lord and Savior. I choose to be engrafted into Christ Jesus. As I receive Jesus, I go from being spiritually dead to being spiritually alive. Being made alive, I now ask to be filled with your Holy Spirit. Holy Spirit, please lead and guide me to all truth. Thank you, Father, for receiving me. Please help me change whatever is in my life that is not your will and does not glorify you. In Jesus's name, I pray, Amen.

I don't spend a lot of time focusing on someone's past; I just like to prepare them for an awesome future in Christ Jesus. Actually, any sin is basically irrelevant other than the sin of not receiving what Jesus did for them (*John 16:9*).

I thoroughly enjoy ushering someone from the kingdom of darkness to the kingdom of light. I know that they will usually be toting a lot of garbage and baggage, but Jesus, in the person of the Holy Spirit, will begin to cleanse them and take them to a place of freedom.

When I minister to someone who doesn't know anything about God and the goodness of God, I love to tell those people testimonies of God's goodness, like the time that He healed Andy's legs and kidneys.

YOUNG MEN RECEIVING JESUS

Being in the restaurant business, I am given the opportunity to interview a lot of people. I have learned to only be led by the Holy Spirit on how to handle situations where people do not know Jesus. Often the Holy Spirit will bring someone to my attention in a very strong way, and I will know that I'm called to minister to them.

On one occasion, a young man whose father had previously worked for me came to interview for a job after his dad had encouraged him to come and talk to me. The parent was concerned because his son was an outspoken atheist, and he was hoping that I could minister to the young man.

The young man was very blunt with me. I remember him saying, "Listen, I know you're a big Christian dude and all that stuff, but I'm not into that and it is not for me. So, if getting this job depends on what I believe, I want no part of it." Well, I assured him that the job was in no way dependent on what he believed; rather, it would be based on how well he worked. He said, "That's cool. Just so we understand each other and you know what I'm about."

Well, with that, the Holy Spirit rose up inside of me, and I said, "I know more about you than you'll ever know." Through the word of knowledge, which is a gift from the Holy Spirit, as mentioned in the 12th chapter of First Corinthians, the Holy Spirit gave me insight into the young man's life. I proceeded to tell him that he was involved in using drugs and in selling drugs. I reminded him that, on at least two different occasions, he faced situations that nearly cost him his life.

After I had finished telling him about his life, which contained information that I would in no way have access to, I proceeded to say, "Now, just so I am sure that we understand each other, you can have the job if you want it, but the job is trivial compared to what is going on in your life. You are being deceived by the devil, held hostage to the work of the enemy. You're in constant torment, and you are risking your life, but the big picture is that, if you die right now, you're going to spend eternity in Hell because you have been living for the enemy instead of receiving what Jesus died to provide for you."

After my little speech, I told him that the interview was over and that now I was going to go over and sit at a nearby picnic table and talk about Jesus. He was welcome to join me if he liked; that way, he could learn how to walk away from all the deception he was living in and receive his salvation through Christ Jesus. Let me just say that I believe he reached the picnic table before I did. He received Jesus and freed himself from all the demonic torment. Now, that's true salvation.

One other time, I had a young man come to Bible study who really wanted to believe in God; however, he just couldn't wrap his head around everything. He had been exposed to so much garbage in his life, been around so many people who talked a good Christian story but failed to walk it out, and was constantly being let down by people.

Again, the Holy Spirit moved upon me to know what to say. I asked him if he would allow one opportunity for the people in Bible study to pray for him so that Jesus could reveal Himself to him, and then he would know whether what I was telling him was true or not.

He let the Bible study group pray for him, and as they laid hands on him, he collapsed on the floor. About a minute later, while regaining his consciousness, he kept calling out Jesus's name. When he was fully revived, he told the group how Jesus encountered him as they prayed for him. He immediately received Jesus and never questioned the existence of God again. Now, that's the goodness of God!

Be led by the Holy Spirit. Don't be satisfied that you still have nine coins— be diligent to seek the one that is lost. Clean up your house and get the clutter out of your life that comes from constantly setting your agenda to the cares of this world. As a result, you will not allow yourself to develop affections for things that have no eternal value.

Constantly live with the revelation that you personally have the opportunity to bring joy to your Heavenly Father when you minister to someone and they choose to be reconciled Back to Him.

Not everyone is going to go to Heaven, and that is not the will of God. Father desires for all to be saved. With that in mind, let's clear up some deception:

1. When I ask someone how they know they're going to Heaven, the response is often, "I'm a good person. I do a lot of good things. I'm a lot better than most people I know." That's great, but that is not going to get you into Heaven. That thought pattern is based on self-righteousness driven by deception from the demonic realm.

   The Scriptures are clear: there is only one way to receive eternal salvation, and that's by receiving Jesus as your Lord and your Savior.

2. Salvation is not received through church membership. Church membership is very important, but salvation must be the result of receiving Jesus as your Lord. You do not get to Heaven by attempting to piggyback off of someone else's salvation; you have to make the decision for yourself.

3. A lot of people are deceived into postponing their salvation until they clean up their act. No, if it were possible to clean up your act on your own, your act would be clean by now. Don't fall for that deception. Receive Jesus, be led by the Holy Spirit, and press into the Word of God to be transformed, that is, to change the way you think so you are able to change the way you behave.

4. When someone has a friend who died and they are grieving for that person, I often approach them and ask if their friend made the decision to receive their salvation through accepting Jesus. If the person has received their salvation, you can grieve for your

loss, but don't grieve for that person—they would not come back even if they could.

People often tell me that they're not sure if the person who died was saved, which I find unsettling. If you are friends with this person, how is it that you never discussed the subject of eternity? People often say, "I don't like to get in people's business." When I hear such a comment, I respond, "If I walk past a burning apartment complex late at night when most people are asleep, and I bang on the doors to wake people up so they can escape the fire, how many people do you think would reprimand me for disturbing them?"

If I had a friend with a child who had wandered off from the parent, that parent would be frantically trying to find the child. How would it be if that friend of mine called me and told me that they needed help searching for the lost child? What would be their response if I told them, "I'm a little busy now, but in a week from Thursday, it might be doable to set aside some time to hunt for your kid." Suffice it to say that the response from my friend would not be very favorable. However, isn't that the kind of response we give to God as He asks us to help find one of His lost kids?

Salvation is huge, so don't take things for granted. Don't let the enemy deceive you. Not everybody is going to enter Heaven when they die. However, you would never know that by attending most funeral services. Did you ever notice that, in a funeral service, the person who has passed away is almost always referred to as now being in Heaven? Sorry, folks, that's not necessarily the case. Everyone attending a funeral always wants to be caring, loving, sensitive, and all that stuff. That's great; however, the lack of truth and honesty could also lure people into a false sense of comfort and security that going to Heaven is a "slam-dunk." The setting of a funeral is a great place to correctly teach the Word of God and offer salvation to the lost.

I would say that many people are not equipped or prepared to minister salvation to someone who has not received Jesus. This is either from a lack of teaching and training or a lack of confidence in their own salvation. A lot of people find it easier to just invite people to church. That's great, but circumstances are not always going to enable you to bring people to church for them to receive what is needed for their lives in that moment. God wants you to be filled with the Holy Spirit, led, guided, and empowered by the Holy Spirit to minister at a moment's notice. Jesus spent most of his ministry time outside the four walls of a church. I believe that we need to receive during a church service to equip us for ministry wherever the Holy Spirit is needed. With that, let's move on to discuss how we receive the Holy Spirit.

Receiving the Holy Spirit

I often hear people say how wonderful it would be to have the opportunity to be with Jesus, just like the disciples did in the earthly ministry of Jesus. I agree that it would be awesome. However, Jesus actually told the disciples that it was better for them if He ascended to be with the Father so that He could send the Holy Spirit and enable them to receive the Holy Spirit so they could actually be filled with the Spirit of God.

The Holy Spirit has the ability to minister through each and every one of us to equip us to walk out the ministry that Jesus modeled for us.

If the enemy can deceive people by convincing them that what they have access to spiritually from our Father is limited, then the responsibility and the revelation of the ministry that we are called to will be limited. If you are not correctly taught and trained in what you have access to, what would ever give you the confidence to minister to the lost in power and authority? The way so many people are trained, they might as well just hide in the corner, hunker down, and pray for daylight!

As soon as I gained revelation of what I was given access to, I realized the magnitude of the responsibility of the ministry that we have been given. When Jesus was baptized in the ministry of John, He rose out of the water and the Holy Spirit descended upon Him. In the fourth chapter of Luke, we are taught that when Jesus received the Holy Spirit, He was filled and controlled by the Holy Spirit. Then the Holy Spirit led Jesus into the wilderness for 40 days. During that time, the Holy Spirit ministered to Jesus, and the Holy Spirit ministered through Jesus. When Jesus came out of the wilderness, the Word says that Jesus was filled with and empowered by the Holy Spirit. When you yield to be filled with the Holy Spirit and controlled by the Holy Spirit, you will not only emerge filled with the Holy Spirit, but also empowered by the Holy Spirit.

Some people always seem to be talking about the wilderness experience that they're going through. If you are going through the wilderness experience that you claim to be going through, you should be prepared to come out of that experience empowered by the Holy Spirit to minister to the oppressed and to the lost, just as Jesus was.

Jesus refers to the Holy Spirit as a spirit of truth, while He also refers to the Holy Spirit as our comforter, counselor, helper, advocate, intercessor, strengthener, and standby. In *Acts 1:8* (AMP), Jesus told the disciples that they would receive power—ability, efficiency, and might—when the Holy Spirit comes upon them, which, in turn, will empower them to be witnesses and live a life that will testify to Jesus. The responsibility is huge, and what we have access to in order to empower us to walk out our responsibility is just as huge. Therefore, we have got to wake up to the revelation that we are empowered by being filled with God Himself. In *Ephesians 3:19 – 20* (AMP), the apostle Paul, by inspiration of the Holy Spirit, reveals to us that we are to be filled with the fullness of God, that we may have the richest measure of the divine presence, and that we become a body wholly filled and flooded with God Himself. Then the apostle Paul goes on to say that because of the power of God that is at work within us, we are able to carry out His purpose and do superabundantly, far over and above all that we may dare ask or think, and even as far as going infinitely beyond our highest prayers, desires, thoughts, and hopes.

No wonder Jesus told us that we need to be prepared to think differently by viewing life and ministry from a kingdom perspective. We have to challenge ourselves to see ministry as more than heading up the church rummage sale, bake sale, and the annual chicken barbecue to raise funds for church repairs. All those activities are good, honorable, and noble, but the person involved in those activities must also walk out the revelation that they are filled with the power and presence of God to minister to the sick and the oppressed, and they must be fully prepared to undo the works of the enemy.

When people are not taught what they have access to, they are not prepared to embrace a ministry that encompasses anything more than what can be accomplished through their own human strength and effort. Unfortunately, the ministry that is restricted to our own strength and effort is not going to correctly and effectively reveal Jesus to the world.

When we are born again, we are blessed with the presence of the Holy Spirit within our spirit. The Holy Spirit is a person with emotions. We are told not to grieve the Holy Spirit, and we are told not to quench the Holy Spirit. I don't believe that the receiving of the Holy Spirit is limited to a one-time event.

On the day of Pentecost, the apostles received the Holy Spirit. However, take a look at the following passage:

> Acts 4:29 – 31 (NKJV): Now, Lord, look on their threats, and grant to Your servants that with all boldness they may speak Your word, 30 by stretching out Your hand to heal, and that signs and wonders may be done through the name of Your holy Servant Jesus."31 And when they had prayed, the place where they were assembled together was shaken; and they were all filled with the Holy Spirit, and they spoke the word of God with boldness.

The religious leaders of the day persecuted the apostles for preaching in the name of Jesus. Instead of backing down, the apostles requested more boldness. It's worth noting that, to equip them with boldness, they asked the Lord that He empower them to minister healing and do signs and wonders in the name of Jesus. When the power of God is displayed to the lost, the Word of God can be preached with all boldness!

Now, notice that, even though they were born again and had already received the Holy Spirit, the Word says, "They were filled with the Holy Spirit."

From the Scriptures, I believe that we receive the Holy Spirit when we receive salvation. However, I believe that as you grow spiritually, the presence of the Holy Spirit within our spirit has the ability to grow and to expand. Limits are never placed and set by the Holy Spirit; any limitation is a result of what we are able to yield to obtain. As we press in to receive more, I believe the Holy Spirit has the ability to continue to increase the impact the Holy Spirit has on our life.

When ministering to people, I have them pray the prayer that I gave you under the section for receiving salvation. I then lay my hands on them and invite the Holy Spirit to fill and flood the spirit of that person receiving salvation. In doing so, I ask the Holy Spirit to allow them to tangibly feel His presence and make them aware of the love that Father has for them.

Deliverance from Mental Torment

For anyone who has suffered through panic disorder, anxiety disorder, or any other kind of tormenting mental oppression, it is some of the worst pain that you can experience. Because of the torment that is involved, I know that the demonic realm is behind any oppression.

Through the journey of my deliverance from panic attacks, through this book, I have given you specific instructions on how to obtain a new mindset, develop new thought patterns, and take demonic thoughts captive to destroy demonic strongholds in your life. All these instructions are based on the Word of God—on the promises of God. If I knew then what I know now, the affliction that I was under would have been short-lived. When God created the Earth, it was devoid of evil. However, when Adam and Eve messed up in the Garden of Eden and the enemy entered in, the knowledge of evil also entered in.

We are a spirit being with a soul, which is comprised of your will, your mind, and your emotions, and the spirit and the soul are housed in a physical body. When someone is under demonic mental torment, the first thing that must happen is for that person to receive their salvation and be filled with the Holy Spirit. I have no interest in merely helping a person attempt to maintain and control mental torment; I want to see it completely driven out of their lives. The demonic realm attacks our mind with thoughts that are evil, tormenting, and oppressive. The battleground is always in the mind.

The work of the enemy is to deceive us to accept incorrect evil thoughts and attempt to cause us to meditate on those thoughts until they cause a pattern of thinking. Once a pattern of thinking is established, thoughts travel the same path, which establishes a stronghold of thinking that embraces fear, depression, and torment. To be free from mental torment, we must learn how to take thoughts captive. Remember, you don't fight thoughts with thoughts; you fight thoughts with words.

The way to obtain your freedom is to speak the promises of God into and over your life. You're going to have to be very selective about what you listen to. Therefore, it is essential that you position yourself to hear the promises of God through CDs and other avenues and that you meditate on the promises of God to begin to break any strongholds. Your key Scripture is the following:

> 2 Corinthians 10:3 – 5 (AMP): For though we walk (live) in the flesh, we are not carrying on our warfare according to the flesh and using mere human weapons. 4 For the weapons of our warfare are not physical [weapons of flesh and blood], but they are mighty before God for the overthrow and destruction of strongholds, 5 [Inasmuch as we] refute arguments and theories and reasonings and every proud and lofty thing that sets itself up against the [true] knowledge of God; and we lead every thought and purpose away captive into the obedience of Christ (the Messiah, the Anointed One).

When I minister to someone who is facing demonic mental torment, it is unlikely that I can simply pray for them and lay my hands on them for them to be granted their freedom. I may have the ability to drive out demonic oppression, but a person has to be responsible to use the Word of God to obtain a sound, healthy mind.

> **2 Timothy 1:7 (NKJV): For God has not given us a spirit of fear, but of power and of love and of a sound mind.**

A person who is facing demonic mental torment has to reestablish the sound mind that God provided them.

When I was being tormented by panic attacks, my mind was anything but healthy and sound. Once I learned the truth of the Word of God, I used the Word of God to change the way I think so that I could think in line with how God thinks; that way, I could easily identify and reject the lies of the enemy.

A person must decide just how badly they desire to be healed and freed from any mental torment. You're going to have to restrict what you listen to and reestablish the way you think. In short, you're going to have to develop a new mindset. All this is accomplished by meditating on the promises of God.

It's very important to not become engaged in strife and unforgiveness.

> **2 Timothy 2:23 – 26 (NKJV): But avoid foolish and ignorant disputes, knowing that they generate strife. 24 And a servant of the Lord must not quarrel but be gentle to all, able to teach, patient, 25 in humility correcting those who are in opposition, if God perhaps will grant them repentance, so that they may know the truth, 26 and that they may come to their senses and escape the snare of the devil, having been taken captive by him to do his will.**

If you enjoy having little spats, arguments, and foolish disputes, get over them and let that junk go. There are many things that open the door for the enemy. Often things that are approved by the world are embraced by God's kids because they are not immediately offensive. The world doesn't view it as being morally wrong, and neither does the believer.

If God says something doesn't work, believe me, it doesn't work. This Scripture says that a person can actually open the door to be taken by the enemy whenever the enemy chooses and to do whatever the enemy wants.

To be healed from demonic mental torment, it is crucial to:

- Allow no unforgiveness.
- Stop petty fights.
- Get rid of the critical spirit. It becomes very easy to criticize when you have no responsibility. Unless you're ministering to someone, mind your own business.
- Don't judge other people.
- Focus on walking in love.

The reason that I'm focusing on behavioral issues first is that it's very important to slam the door on any activities in your life that give the demonic realm access through your disobedience.

Now, ways to obtain your deliverance:

- Quit speaking words that reinforce and empower the enemy. Quit saying that things drive you crazy, that you hit your limit, that you can't take certain things anymore, etc.
- Go to the Word of God, find the promises of God that relate to obtaining a strong, healthy mind, and continually speak them over your life.
- When you have an incorrect thought, immediately use the name of Jesus and take authority over that thought and cast it out. I simply say *to* myself: *That thought is not of God, and I reject that thought in the name of Jesus.*
- Train yourself to focus on the positive and resist dwelling on the negative.

> Philippians 4:8 – 9 (NKJV): 8 Finally, brethren, whatever things are true, whatever things are noble, whatever things are just, whatever things are pure, whatever things are lovely, whatever things are of good report, if there is any virtue and if there is anything praiseworthy—meditate on these things. 9 The things which you learned and received and heard and saw in me, these do, and the God of peace will be with you.

PHYSICAL HEALING

The amount of confusion there is over the will of God for people to be healed physically never fails to amaze me. Anytime that you see the degree of confusion there is over a matter such as physical healing, we must be aware that what we are pressing in for is a potential threat to the demonic realm.

> James 3:13 – 17 (NKJV): Who is wise and understanding among you? Let him show by good conduct that his works are done in the meekness of wisdom. 14 But if you have bitter envy and self-seeking in your hearts, do not boast and lie against the truth. 15 This wisdom does not descend from above, but is earthly, sensual, demonic. 16 For where envy and self-seeking exist, confusion and every evil thing are there. 17 But the wisdom that is from above is first pure, then peaceable, gentle, willing to yield, full of mercy and good fruits, without partiality and without hypocrisy.

Not everyone I have ever ministered to for physical healing has received their healing. That does not change the truth that it is God's desire for people to be healed physically and that Jesus died on the cross for them to obtain their physical healing.

Not everyone that I have ever ministered to for salvation has received their salvation; however, this does not change the truth that it is God's desire for all to be saved.

Too many times, doctrines have been allowed to be established to try to answer questions that we are not in the position to receive answers for. We are in a war; therefore, we have opposition. The demonic realm attempts to block what we have the ability to receive from our Father and from the Kingdom of God.

Let's first examine the truth about healing:

- Jesus spent over half of His earthly ministry ministering physical healing to people.
- Jesus healed everyone who positioned themselves to be healed.
- Jesus healed multitudes of people.
- Jesus sent the apostles and the disciples out to minister healing to people.
- Jesus commissioned the Church to continue the earthly ministry that He modeled after He was raised from the dead and ascended to Heaven.
- When Jesus was lashed 39 times, the Bible notes, *"By the stripes of Jesus, we are healed."*
- Jesus never told anyone that God made them sick.
- Jesus never told anyone that they could not be healed because it was the will of God that they remain sick.
- Jesus never put sickness on anyone to enable them to become closer to God.

As soon as the apostles were filled with the Holy Spirit, they started ministering to people. One of the first records of the ministry of Peter and John was the healing of the lame man in the third chapter of Acts.

There are two events in the Bible that seem to trip people up in terms of God's will for people to be healed.

First, in the Old Testament, there was a man named Job. God referred to Job as one of the most upright and reverent men on Earth. If you have questions about the life of Job, I suggest that you read the book of Job.

As it is taught, Satan challenged God to allow him to bring harm upon the life of Job to prove that Job would curse God if evil came upon him. Job persevered and did not curse God.

I believe that Satan's inability to cause a man to curse God really started to weaken the hold that the enemy had on mankind because it revealed that mankind could actually remain strong and honor God.

Here, I would like to mention a few a points:

- This story is an account in the Old Testament, under an inferior covenant.
- Jesus never mentioned the account of Job during His earthly ministry.
- The account of Job is often taught in a way that makes one believe that Job went through testing and trials most of his life. Biblical historians, however, refer to the event of the trial as being less than one year in duration.
- Before Satan attacked Job, he was the richest man in that area. After Satan's attack and when Job remained honorable to God, God blessed him by giving him double of everything he had before.
- If you're going to claim to be tested and tried like Job, the story needs to end with you emerging victorious and being blessed with double of what you began with.
- The second event is in *2 Corinthians 12:7 – 9*, where Paul refers to having a thorn in his flesh. Paul tells a story that God enabled him to experience Heaven. So that Paul would not be prideful, he received a thorn in the flesh.
- God gave Paul the opportunity to experience Heaven.
- To keep Paul from being exalted, he received a thorn in the flesh.
- The Word of God does not say that the thorn in the flesh was sickness.
- The Word of God does not say that God gave Paul the thorn in the flesh.

- The Word of God says that the thorn in the flesh was a messenger of Satan.
- Paul asked God to cause the thorn in the flesh to leave him.
- God told Paul that His grace was sufficient for Paul. The question comes in whether the grace was to endure the affliction or to empower Paul to rid himself of the affliction. The Word of God says that Grace is a gift from God through Jesus. The word "grace," as used in the Scriptures, primarily refers to enabling power and spiritual healing offered through the mercy and love of Jesus Christ. Grace means unmerited and undeserved favor.

My question is that, since Jesus gave us the power, authority, and responsibility to undo the works of the enemy, was this something that Paul should be praying to God about? If so, how should Paul have dealt with using Jesus's name?

I bring these two scriptural references to you not to entice some sort of debate over them but rather to educate you enough to press in for yourself to study the Scriptures.

Through studying the Scriptures, focusing in on the earthly ministry of Jesus, I am convinced that it's the will of God for all people to be healed. I believe the reason why there is so much confusion over the matter is that the demonic realm works very hard to restrict any power and authority that is accomplished through the faith of the believers.

As we read before, the demonic realm worked behind incorrect religious teaching to try to put an end to preaching in the name of Jesus. We studied those Scriptures in the third and fourth chapter of the book of Acts. When I minister to someone in the name of Jesus and they receive their healing, like in the case of Andy, when he received healing for his kidneys and his legs after the doctors had told him that there was no chance for him to be healed, it reveals the goodness of our Father God to the world, and it also reveals how our God is the one true God.

As we learn from the Scriptures about how to obtain healing, it is very important that you are convinced that physical healing is the will of God.

We have an enemy, and that enemy is the demonic realm. Therefore, we have to be able to stand our ground in faith in order to receive from the Kingdom of God while we are in this earthly hostile environment.

Because I know that Jesus died on the cross to bless us with the access to physical healing, when I minister to people to receive their healing, I speak declarations of faith from the Scriptures in the name of Jesus. The time that I spend in prayer with my Father is a time of continually building my relationship with Him to understand His heart for people and to receive any specific instructions or assignments He may have for me.

For myself, I know I need to continually increase the time that I spend in prayer with my Father. It is so easy getting caught up in the busyness of the world and, all of a sudden, find that you've just run out of time for the things that should be top priority. Time spent with my Father blesses me with the confidence to walk out the power and authority that He provided me to effectively minister with.

Over the years, I have really grown to understand how much love our Father has for people. I want to position myself to allow His love to flow through me to impact the people that He wants to minister to. In ministering physical healing to people:

1. I never question whether it's God's will or not for someone to be healed. I know the heart of my Father.
2. God ministers through me in the person of Holy Spirit. I can't heal people. I can only allow the One who can heal people to minister through me.
3. I position myself to be led by the Holy Spirit to listen for instructions. I don't hear God with an audible voice; I hear the voice of my Father in my spirit through promptings and a sense of knowing.
4. Sometimes the Holy Spirit guides me to first minister salvation and then physical healing, though physical healing can occasionally come first.

5. I spend time with a person to teach them the heart of my Father so they have the confidence to believe and are in a position to receive.

6. You have to discern between facts and truth. When someone has an obvious physical ailment, that is a fact. However, the truth of the Word of God has the ability to override that fact. I look at all facts as temporary, and I look at truth as eternal. The reason I mention this is because, after I minister healing to someone, I need them to confess that they are healed in the name of Jesus. That is truth. The truth is that they are healed. The fact is that they may still have symptoms; however, this is okay because the truth will correct the facts. It is very important to speak truth in line with what you believe in.

7. I do not discourage people from going to see the doctor or taking medication. However, I always encourage them to see a doctor or take medications by faith, and also to believe that God will be the one that ultimately heals them.

8. I don't always pray for people immediately. Sometimes the Holy Spirit will lead me to spend time in prayer for that person and for myself to position me to more effectively receive from Father and the provisions of His kingdom.

9. It is often the case that, when I minister to people for them to receive healing from Father, I will speak the desired result over that person in the name of Jesus, and then I will lay hands on them. In studying the Scriptures, this is often what Jesus modeled for us during His earthly ministry.

10. I don't focus on the problem or the severity of the illness. I want to be moved by what I believe, not by what I see. Often I will intentionally not allow myself to hear all the gory details of the severity of the illness. All of that information is irrelevant to them receiving from the Kingdom of God. I don't want to be moved by circumstances.

11. Along with not wanting to be moved by circumstances, not everyone that you minister to will be healed immediately. We studied about seed, time, harvest. I will speak the name of Jesus over a person and declare their healing, while I will also instruct

that person to continually call themselves healed in the name of Jesus and to continually thank God for their healing.

I can't allow myself to be moved by what I see, I can't be moved by what I feel, I can't be moved by circumstances, and I can't be moved by any fear and doubt. I can only allow myself to be moved by what I believe.

DRIVING OUT
FIBROMYALGIA
KRISTINA'S MIRACLE

One of my employees, Kristina, had fibromyalgia when I hired her. She found that she could not physically handle the job because of the effects of the illness. Upon hearing this, I suggested the following to Kristina: "Why don't we just drive that fibromyalgia out of you, and then you can get on with life." She was a strong believer in God, so I knew we were in a great position to receive. In the name of Jesus, I spoke to the fibromyalgia to make a quick exit, and I demanded perfect healing for her body.

This is important: the healing did not manifest itself immediately, but she did receive it immediately by faith. Amazingly, within a day or two, she was completely healed of a disease that had kept her debilitated for over six years.

CASTING OUT DEMONS

It's interesting that in the earthly ministry of Jesus, He spent a large percent of His time casting out demons and healing the sick. Why is it that demons are not cast out? Is it because they are no longer in opposition to us? Absolutely not, or at least, not according to the Scriptures.

The reason we do not see people cast out demons and laying hands on the sick to enable them to recover is that most churches do not teach, train, and equip people for the ministry that Jesus and the apostles displayed for us. Remember, Jesus said that the person who has seen Him has correctly seen the Father. Jesus also said that it is the Father within Him—the Father does the work.

So, what happened? Did God lose His focus all of a sudden? Absolutely not. We are filled with the Holy Spirit to be empowered to undo the works of the enemy.

It's amazing that, in most churches, the demonic realm is never even mentioned. The demonic realm is the enemy of the Church, so I would think that would make it kind of a priority to minister about and to train the congregation on how to drive out demons and minister health and healing to the sick. Is it that the Church has become so civilized and so conformed to the world that the thought of driving out a demon is just too much to embrace?

In *Luke 4:1 – 12*, we see that Jesus was led by the Holy Spirit into the wilderness to face the devil. Jesus entered the wilderness full of and controlled by the Holy Spirit, and He came out of the wilderness filled with and under the power of the Holy Spirit. We will pick up this teaching in verse 13.

> Luke 4:13 – 14 (AMP): And when the devil had ended every [the complete cycle of] temptation, he [temporarily] left Him [that is, stood off from Him] until another more opportune and favorable time. 14 Then Jesus went back full of and under the power of the [Holy] Spirit into Galilee, and the fame of Him spread through the whole region round about.

It is interesting that it says that the devil exposed Jesus to a complete cycle of temptation. Despite the fact that Jesus remained strong and resisted the devil, the devil did not give up and kept watching for a more opportune time.

> Luke 4:14 – 19 (AMP): Then Jesus went back full of and under the power of the [Holy] Spirit into Galilee, and the fame of Him spread through the whole region round about. 15 And He Himself conducted [a course of] teaching in their synagogues, being recognized and honored and praised by all. 16 So He came to Nazareth, [that Nazareth] where He had been brought up, and He entered the synagogue, as was His custom on the Sabbath day. And He stood up to read. 17 And there was handed to Him [the roll of] the book of the prophet Isaiah. He opened (unrolled) the book and found the place where it was written, 18 The Spirit of the Lord [is] upon Me, because He has anointed Me [the Anointed One, the Messiah] to preach the good news (the Gospel) to the poor; He has sent Me to announce release to the captives and recovery of sight to the blind, to send forth as delivered those who are oppressed [who are downtrodden, bruised, crushed, and broken down by calamity], 19 To proclaim the accepted and acceptable year of the Lord [the day when salvation and the free favors of God profusely abound].

Jesus was fully empowered by the Holy Spirit. The Holy Spirit empowered Jesus to undo the works of the enemy; that is, to preach to the poor, set the captives free, bring sight to the blind, and deliver those who are oppressed.

This was the work of Father in the person of the Holy Spirit ministering through Jesus. Take a look at the priorities. Everything was geared to undo the works of the enemy. Why is this not preached today with the same urgency and preciseness? It's because the enemy works very hard through deception to keep the sons and daughters of Father from knowing who they are, the ministry that they are called to, and the power and authority that is made available to them.

> Luke 4:31 – 37 (AMP): Then He went down to Capernaum, a city of Galilee, and was teaching them on the Sabbaths. 32 And they were astonished at His teaching, for His word was with authority. 33 Now in the synagogue there was a man who had a spirit of an unclean demon. And he cried out with a loud voice, 34 saying, "Let us alone! What have we to do with You, Jesus of Nazareth? Did You come to destroy us? I know who You are—the Holy One of God!" 35 But Jesus rebuked him, saying, "Be quiet, and come out of him!" And when the demon had thrown him in their midst, it came out of him and did not hurt him. 36 Then they were all amazed and spoke among themselves, saying, "What a word this is! For with authority and power He commands the unclean spirits, and they come out." 37 And the report about Him went out into every place in the surrounding region.

This is very important because Jesus entered the synagogue and found a man there who had a spirit of an unclean demon. Look at what the demon said: "Did you come to destroy us? I know who you are."

Isn't that interesting? How did this demon know about Jesus? Well, the demonic realm watched their boss, Satan, get beaten up by Jesus in the wilderness. Verse 14 says that the fame of Jesus went out through all the surrounding regions. His fame did not just reach the people; his fame was experienced by the demonic realm because, for the first time since the fall of mankind in the Garden of Eden, a man could be spiritually alive, filled with the Holy Spirit, and, therefore, be empowered to undo the works of Satan and all his demons.

As recorded *Luke 9-10,* Jesus sent the disciples out to preach the Kingdom of God and display the Kingdom of God in power. Jesus commanded the disciples to preach the Kingdom of God, heal the sick, and drive out demons.

In *Luke 10:17 – 20*, the Scriptures record that Jesus commissioned 70 of His followers, along with His 12 disciples, to preach and minister the Kingdom of God. The 70 returned with excitement, proclaiming that even the demons were subject to them as they used the name of Jesus. He then proceeded to tell them that He had given them the authority and power to trample upon serpents and scorpions and over all the power of the enemy. Then He goes on to say, *"Do not rejoice in this, that the demons are subject to you, but rejoice that your names are written in heaven."*

Jesus provided the disciples with a very valuable concept concerning ministry. Ministry on this Earth involves inviting the Kingdom of God into a hostile environment of this world system. There is always the potential to face disappointments and setbacks in the midst of obtaining spiritual victories. Since not all of our questions are always going to be answered, we must be prepared for that reality. We build our lives on the foundation of faith in Jesus Christ. We prepare for a successful ministry through the determination to not be moved by what we see and the determination to remain steadfastly prepared to patiently endure. Here, what Jesus is teaching us is that, to be successful, you must protect your joy, and the ultimate joy is the revelation that, no matter what we face, our names are written in the Lamb's book of life and that we are going to spend eternity with Jesus and our Father. Joy is an extremely valuable spiritual force.

Having said that, if you're going to walk out the ministry that Holy Spirit guides you through, you're going to most likely face people who are either harassed by the enemy, oppressed by the enemy, or even possessed by the enemy. In *Matthew 12:28* (NKJV), Jesus gives us the revelation about spiritual warfare as he tells us, *"But if I cast out demons by the Spirit of God, surely the kingdom of God has come upon you."*

If you are born again and you are filled with the Holy Spirit, you are empowered to set the captives free, and you are empowered to drive out demons. To do so, you must know who you are in Christ Jesus. Demons have the potential to bring about ugly manifestations. Demons do this in an attempt to get your eyes off of Jesus and onto the situation that they create.

I remember casting out a demon from a man who was so empowered by it that it took four people to hold him down while I sat on his chest and drove it out. While casting out a demon from a girl, it actually caused her to bounce off the floor as she lay on her back.

As you face the demonic realm, try to take your eyes off the situation, take your eyes off yourself, and realize that you are empowered by the presence of the Holy Spirit residing in your born-again spirit. Demons are not intimidated by the volume of your voice or shouts of determination. When casting out demons, be led by the Holy Spirit and be very grounded by who you are in Christ Jesus. Be prepared for the unexpected.

Demons will always attempt to catch you off guard in order to generate fear. They are empowered through deception, and they are empowered through fear. Isn't it interesting that fear and deception are the major components of panic attacks and anxiety disorder?

As you study the account of the demon-possessed man in the country of the Gadarenes, notice that, even though the man was possessed by more than a thousand demons, he was still able to approach Jesus and worship Him. That goes to show how important it is to have the confidence that we can stay true to God in the midst of any demonic attacks

Walk free from deception and make a stance of faith that refuses to entertain fear. You cast demons out by the revelation of your relationship with Father through your Lord Jesus Christ, and you are empowered by the infilling of the Holy Spirit.

THE END OF THE LINE

Well, we have come to the end of the two journeys.

Being a former victim of panic attacks and anxiety disorder, I just want to reveal to you just how amazing it is to be free from panic attacks and from the torment of excessive anxiety. I also want you to have the confidence that you can also be free from any mental torment that you are facing.

During the time that I was held hostage by panic attacks, I could not find a way out. Well, I broke free and I am confident that you also can obtain your freedom. The desire of my heart is that you are able to use all the information that I have provided in order to obtain your path of escape.

Ultimately, I know it was my faith in God that brought about my freedom. What was so awesome about the two journeys that I traveled was that I obtained freedom from my panic attacks; however, even more importantly, I also obtained freedom from the confusion in the world relating to the existence of God as I obtained the revelation of His nature as well as His will and purpose for my life.

God has provided everything that we need to obtain our freedom from the enemy and the evil in the world. God sent His Son—Jesus—to undo the works of the enemy and to enable us to be reconciled back to our Father God.

If you're going to walk in freedom, you need the revelation that there is a demonic realm that operates for no other reason than to attempt to cause death, loss, and destruction in your life—*John 10:10*. Unfortunately, too many churches have strayed away from the accurate teaching of the demonic realm; and therefore, people are held hostage through their ignorance.

> **Hebrews 2:14 – 15 (AMP): Since, therefore, [these His] children share in flesh and blood [in the physical nature of human beings], He [Himself] in a similar manner partook of the same [nature], that by [going through] death He might bring to naught and make of no effect him who had the power of death—that is, the devil—15 And also that He might deliver and completely set free all those who through the [haunting] fear of death were held in bondage throughout the whole course of their lives.**

It is so pivotal that you receive the revelation of this Scripture. This passage is giving us the revelation that Jesus had to take on the same nature as mankind. Jesus had to take on a physical body to enable Him to retrieve what was lost in the fall of man in the Garden of Eden.

Jesus destroyed the works of the enemy by empowering us to be engrafted into Him, thus, enabling us to be filled with the Holy Spirit.

Jesus revealed the nature of God, and He died to empower us to walk out the will of our Father. When we are filled with the Holy Spirit, we are empowered to successfully do warfare against the demonic realm. Not only that, but Jesus also blessed us with access to eternal life so that we never again have to fear death.

If you are going to walk free from panic or anxiety disorder, you must embrace this passage in Hebrews, along with many other passages in the Word of God that can drive out deception and set you free.

Obtaining freedom from fear will enable you to disarm the onslaught of a panic attack.

By being engrafted into Jesus Christ, learning how to be free from the cares of this world will, in turn, free us from that which causes anxiety disorder.

We have an enemy—the demonic realm. Jesus defeated the demonic realm, and then He blessed us with the use of His name to reinforce the defeat of the demonic realm.

I'm going to conclude our journeys by providing insight into how to live above the evil in this world, and I'm also going to give you some nuggets of spiritual insight into how to protect the way you think.

STUPID, HUNGRY FISH

We were made in the image and likeness of God. Within each one of us is a cry to be united to our Creator—Father God. Since we were created to enter into a relationship with our Father, when we are not in that relationship and fulfilled and satisfied by that relationship, there is going to be a void.

The reason the enemy is so successful in destroying the lives of people is that they have voids in their lives. When people are not engrafted into Jesus Christ and fail to walk in the correct revelation of their Father, a huge void is created in their lives because of the lack of relationship they have with Father God, which causes an identity crisis and lack of purpose. When there is a lack of a correct relationship with Father God, people are forced to go to the world to attempt to obtain their purpose and their identity. This puts people in a position where they are very vulnerable to the demonic realm.

When I go fishing, I often go to a stream that is filled with stupid, hungry fish. I want to find fish that are searching for something. I want them to be too stupid to identify that the bait that I am presenting to them will ultimately cause them to be captured by the hook that is covered by that alluring bait. When I am fishing, I want the fish to be naïve and vulnerable due to their hunger. This is exactly the condition the enemy desires to find in mankind. The devil wants us to be stupid and very hungry.

Our stupidity is created by incorrect religious teachings that have the effect of making us increasingly vulnerable to the attacks of the enemy.

Our hunger is created out of our lack of relationship with our Father God, which will result in creating a void. The void is created by the lack of a relationship of who we are in the eyes of our Father and the purpose that we are called to.

Sorry for being so blunt, but what incorrect religious teaching, along with misappropriated false humility, has achieved is to make us vulnerable, to make us stupid, hungry men and women.

The enemy wants us to be an easy target for his deception. The enemy wants us to be unskillful in the word of righteousness—*Hebrews 5:13*—so that we are ignorant and ineffective in spiritual warfare. The enemy wants us to be hungry as a result of the lack of a relationship with our Father, which thus causes a void in our lives and confusion over our purpose.

In *James 4:7*, the Word says that we are to resist the devil and the devil will flee from us. Unfortunately, too many Christians are ignorant of the ways of the demonic realm. So often do I hear people complaining that they are getting beaten up by the devil; the solution to their problem is simple: you have not been resisting the devil. On the other hand, how can someone resist what they have never been correctly taught actually exists, and who have not been taught how to effectively do spiritual warfare.

In *1 Peter 5:8*, the Word says that our adversary, the devil, goes around like a roaring lion seeking out those whom he can destroy. You need this revelation! The enemy is *like* a roaring lion, but is not truly a roaring lion. The enemy attempts to deceive you into thinking that he is as powerful as a roaring lion when, basically, we have the spiritual weapons and authority to reduce him into a timid kitten. Again, it's an issue of incorrect teaching. Instead of driving the devil out, people flee from the enemy because they do not understand that they are facing a roar that has no bite to back it up.

In the world, a successful thief is one who is able to go undetected and or one who can operate in a way that makes someone else look responsible for any losses. This is accomplished through deception. The enemy works through an incorrect religious mindset to promote the type of smokescreen that he can hide behind.

Jesus came to reveal the nature of our Father. Jesus made the declaration that, if we have correctly seen Him, then we have correctly seen the Father. Never once did Jesus make someone sick, cause someone to be sick, nor promote sickness as an avenue for a person to enable them to come to know Him better. Never once did Jesus put his blessing upon a natural storm to cause destruction.

Either the devil needs to be commended for his amazing ability to deceive us or we need to begin to take responsibility for allowing the Father to be revealed incorrectly.

Because we have not walked out the ministry that Jesus modeled for us, we have opened the door to the enemy to deceive churches, and, therefore, make us ineffective in the ministry that Jesus gave us to reconcile the lost back to Father.

The insurance company puts disclaimers in their policies that they do not cover damage done by an "act of God." Where did this language come from? It came from the world, with the support of churches that are filled with people who, unfortunately, do not know the nature of our Father God.

The enemy has established a perfect set up. The enemy causes death, loss, and destruction, and through deception, the enemy deceives churches into promoting these demonic activities as being initiated and authorized by God. The same God that is being preached from many church pulpits is not the God that Jesus revealed through His earthly ministry. Even though this country was founded on the revelation of God, we have allowed that revelation to slip away. We have allowed God to be pushed out of the classroom, and we have allowed His name to be associated with demonic activities, such as sickness and natural disasters. Because of this, many people have turned away from God. In doing so, the void in a person's life is left unfulfilled; therefore, people are deceived into attempting to go to the world to receive that which is only available from Father God.

In the restaurant business, we employ quite a large number of young men and women. I am amazed at how many of them come from broken families. The majority do not know God, so they live a life that is devoid of their crucial relationship with God. So many young people today are held hostage by an orphan spirit, which makes them feel inferior, out of place, unwanted, and with no purpose.

It is time for people to step up and demand that the authentic Gospel of Jesus Christ be preached and preached correctly.

As I minister to people, I find that I'm led by the Holy Spirit to teach and train people to obtain their relationship with God as His son/daughter, to obtain their identity as being in Christ Jesus, and to obtain the revelation that they have a purpose in this life on Earth.

When Jesus was baptized, the Holy Spirit descended upon Him, and a voice came from Heaven, saying, *"You are my beloved Son; in You, I am well pleased."*

It's interesting to note that, after Jesus received validation from God, He entered the wilderness and was tempted by the devil. The very first thing that the enemy attacked Jesus with was His relationship with God and His identity. The attack of the enemy came in the form of a question: *"If you are the Son of God, command this stone to become bread."*

The temptation was to get Jesus to question His identity. Jesus was tempted by the enemy and came out victorious. The victory of Jesus was obtained because He knew the relationship that He had with God; therefore, He knew His identity as being the Son of God, and He also knew His purpose.

In defeating the panic attacks in my life, it was crucial that I understood that I was in a relationship with Father and I was His son. I also received the revelation that my purpose was to minister to the lost and to those who were held hostage by mental torment.

I never once questioned that God was the author of my panic attacks. I knew the attack was from the demonic realm. I also knew God to be my Father, and I looked to my Father to find my way of escape. My way of escape came from Scriptures such as the following:

> **Colossians 3:1 – 3 (NKJV): If then you were raised with Christ, seek those things which are above, where Christ is, sitting at the right hand of God. 2 Set your mind on things above, not on things on the earth. 3 For you died, and your life is hidden with Christ in God.**

Through this and other Scriptures, I obtained the revelation of my relationship with God, my identity as being in Christ Jesus, and my purpose of revealing Jesus to the lost.

It's crucial for you to obtain revelation of your relationship, identity, and purpose.

The years before, during, and after being held hostage to panic attacks, I learned to live with a kingdom perspective, I learned to gain the revelation of not to focus on things on the Earth but instead set my mind on the things that are above.

As I took you on the journey of the years that I dealt with panic attacks, I gave you information on how to defeat panic attacks using godly principles. We learned how to put a stop to fear, and we learned how to develop a new mindset. We also learned how to take demonic thoughts captive to the obedience of Christ.

No matter what you are battling with, no matter what you are being held hostage to, your answer and deliverance are found by not focusing on yourself but by walking out the revelation that you are engrafted into Christ Jesus. To die to yourself means that you look to God to obtain your relationship, your identity, and your purpose. I yield to the Holy Spirit to cause me to be transformed and to enable me to walk out the ministry that Jesus died to equip me for.

Every born-again, spirit-filled son or daughter of God has a ministry. The ministry is to reconcile the lost back to Father and to undo the works of the enemy.

When I go fishing, I like to fish in a place where the fish are hungry and stupid. However, when I walk out my life in Christ Jesus, I want my relationship with Father to take away any hunger and I want the revelation that the Holy Spirit provides to keep me from being stupid.

The enemy can't destroy you; the enemy must get you to self-destruct. The enemy wants you hungry and stupid. The enemy wants to lay out the bait in anticipation that you will fall for the trap that he has set. The enemy wants you very discontent so that he can draw you into making impulsive, harmful decisions.

The contentment in my life comes from the foundation built upon my relationship with God, my identity as being in Christ Jesus, and my purpose of ministering to the lost. This minimizes the chance that I will make impulsive and harmful decisions.

Do I still make mistakes? Most certainly, but through a dependency on the Holy Spirit, they continue to be fewer and fewer. There will always be a tendency to be drawn to harmful behavior and to have affections for things in the world. However, I've learned through dependency on the Holy Spirit that I can continually raise the standard that I live by.

Within the contents of this book, I mainly focused on being delivered from panic attacks. However, the spiritual principles that I provided for you have the potential to offer freedom from anxiety, mental torment, alcoholism, drug abuse, and anything else that attacks your flesh to make you a hostage to the demonic realm and ineffective in walking out the purpose of your life.

Whatever you are struggling with, continue to minimize the effects of the addictions and other demonic attacks by increasing the revelation of your spiritual **relationship, identity,** and **purpose.** To make it easy to remember, I like to refer to it as **R.I.P.**

Any time I face opposition from the enemy through temptations to enter into incorrect behavior, I ask myself if that behavior matches the revelation of who I am in Christ Jesus. As you learn to yield to the guidance of the Holy Spirit and continue to increase the revelation that you are engrafted into Jesus Christ, junk from the world and opposition from the demonic realm will begin to drop off of you, allowing you to find your freedom.

Remember, the Word says that as we resist the enemy, the enemy flees from us. Don't be deceived into allowing the enemy to cause you to set your eyes on yourself and your problems instead of fixing your focus on being one with Christ Jesus.

If you want your freedom, you're going to have to fight for it. The way you engage in a fight successfully is to remember that your warfare is directed at the demonic realm, not people. You do warfare by yielding to allow the Holy Spirit to minister through you in power and authority.

Jesus obtained the victory for us, so we don't fight for a place of victory— we fight from a place of victory. We reinforce the defeat of the enemy by reinforcing our stance of victory in Christ Jesus.

Don't be deceived into allowing yourself to fall into self-pity. Self-pity does nothing but force you to look at yourself and away from Jesus. Let me tell you a little bit about self-pity.

Self-pity is the Taj Mahal of negativity. Even if you do not impose self-pity on yourself, if you surround yourself with family, friends, social media, and a negative environment, the door to self-pity is opened to demonic deception. You must remove yourself from negative people and situations if you are serious about regaining your life.

There will always be opposition and roadblocks that you will need to steer clear of. There will always be stumbling blocks, such as fear and the opportunity to fall into offense. The world will always attempt to cause detours. There will be potholes that you will need to navigate around, and there will be distractions that you need to resist.

No matter what the obstacle, you now know that you will never be alone—your Heavenly Father never abandons us. Although we may turn from Him, He is always there waiting with outstretched arms. Copy this and carry this in your pocket and refer to it when needed.

> **The pain that you've been feeling can't compare with the joy that's coming!**

This is from *Romans 8:18*. Copy it, carry it with you, and read it whenever you encounter any opposition.

If you desire complete freedom, peace, joy, and contentment, evaluate the quality of your life. What do you find? Is it where you want to be? What are you being held hostage to? Do you find yourself in the same dilemma that I was in before I made a commitment to obtain what I knew was available?

I was successful and have shared with you what worked for me. Many whom I have counseled have also been set free. It is now your time.

Be determined. Be relentless.

You have everything it takes to succeed, build mental barriers, capture runaway thoughts, and gain back what you have lost because you now have the tools and know you are not alone. Demand of yourself to be who God created you to be. Allow the Holy Spirit to be your navigator and let your love for God and for others be your motivator. Jesus already blazed the trail—all you need to do is allow the Holy Spirit to guide you the way Jesus did.

You are now armed to be able to resist compromise, excuses, and any justification for potential failure. Freedom and abundant life are waiting for you at the completion of your journey.

You are blessed with the opportunity to overcome all self-pity and self-doubt to be filled with the Holy Spirit and become a new creation. Allow the Holy Spirit to lead and guide you to all truth and to obtain a Kingdom of God perspective.

You were created for victory.
Praying for your deliverance.

A MESSAGE FORM PASTOR BRANDON STOLTZFUS FROM UGANDA

I have known Brian for over 12 years; I first met him as he led a Bible study for young adults. My first night at the Bible study changed my life! I was filled with Holy Spirit that night and experienced a miracle that repaired my ears from hearing loss and constant drainage. When I turned 18, Brian became my mentor and spiritual father. Over the past 12 years, I have learned from Brian more things than a book can hold. He is the best counselor, teacher, and friend that I have ever known, and I have witnessed Brian counseling people through panic attack, demonic oppression, and addiction. I personally have witnessed and experienced countless miracles as I have spent time with Brian. He has impacted thousands of people with his ability to teach and equip them to live out what God has enabled them to live out.

My name is Brandon Stoltzfus and I am currently living in Masaka, Uganda with my beautiful wife and three babies! We are so thankful for Brian as he is like family. So much of who I am today is because of all that Brian has poured into me. We love Jesus so very much and we live to reveal the truth of Jesus to anyone.

Brandon and Jennika Stoltzfus are assistant directors for abandoned and orphaned children - Love and Care for All Uganda https://loveandcareforall. org/about-us/. *We currently have about 106 children. Brandon is serving as pastor for Mission Assistance International, a non-profit sending, equipping, and supporting ministry in foreign missions.* www.missionassist.org.

Some of the proceeds from this book go to support ministry outreach in Africa and Haiti.

ENDORSEMENTS

I have suffered with mild to severe anxiety most of my life. After reading this book, I have learned new ways to quiet my mind and guide my thoughts into new patterns of thinking. We so quickly give up on trusting God, this book explains how to use His power to obtain freedom.

Jean Kelley, retired teacher, mother and worrier.

Brian, you have written a wonderful book—it has an important message that is well communicated, with clear steps on how to use your ideas. You've done a particularly good job of providing direct support from Scripture for your techniques and ideas—there are a huge number of passages that speak directly to the subject at hand, lending great weight to what you are saying. I also think that when a passage from Scripture does not directly address the ideas presented, you've done an excellent job of connecting the dots for the reader.

Jefferson, Primary Editor, FirstEditing

I have had the esteemed privilege of working for Brian Ludwig for nearly 11 years. Over those years I have witnessed many set free from panic and anxiety. In Sept 2008, Brian prayed over me and Jesus Christ healed me of fibromyalgia. I had been so ill that my doctor told me I would surely die. Chapter by chapter, I read the manuscript as it was being written. I have no doubt that this book will change lives and light a path for people who are seeking our Lord and Savior Jesus Christ. Brian's experiences and testimonies in this book will serve as a ministry to the lost.

Kristina Rineer, employee, received my healing in 2008

Brian, I have to say that I actually learned a lot from reading this book, and I have been thinking about some of your tips recently! You wrote in a straightforward and informal manner, which will help the reader connect with you. I felt that you used real-life examples and spoke in a way that was not overly academic in nature. This made the information easier to understand and apply to the reader's daily life, step by step.

Max, Assistant Editor, FirstEditing

The Author does a good job explaining panic attacks from the patient's point of view. Along the way he provides hope and encouragement using both effective medical treatment and self-help. He also offers Christian spiritual insight as another avenue for help for those suffering from this challenging illness.

Charles Lowe MD

It was a privilege to read about how Brian has overcome his own trials and now uses what he has learned to minister to others. He infuses his humor, wisdom, and deep faith into this informative book, which is aimed at helping others find freedom. Even if you are not struggling with panic attacks, you will find great information to apply to your life. I look forward to seeing what else God lays on his heart to share!

Allie Swann, friend, proofreader

CONTACT INFORMATION

ASK the AUTHOR
Visit our website to find out how.

seekingpeaceandjoy.com

9 781973 665977